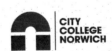

# FOOD SOLUTIONS
# Irritable bowel syndrome

## Recipes and Advice to Control Symptoms

### Patsy Westcott

hamlyn

**SAFETY NOTE**

This book should not be considered a replacement for professional medical treament. A doctor should be consulted in all matters relating to health, particularly in respect of any symptoms which may require diagnosis or medical attention. While the advice and information in this book are believed to be accurate, neither the author nor the publisher can accept any legal responsibility for any injury or illness sustained while following the treatments and diet plan.

First published in Great Britain in 2002 by
Hamlyn, a division of Octopus Publishing Group Ltd
2–4 Heron Quays, London E14 4JP

This revised edition published 2004

ISBN 0 600 61059 4

A CIP catalogue record for this book is available from the British Library

Printed and bound in the United Kingdom by the Mackays of Chatham

10  9  8  7  6  5  4  3  2  1

# Contents

# Introduction

Irritable bowel syndrome, or IBS as it is usually known, is one of the most common digestive disorders in the industrialized world. It is also one of the most puzzling. IBS affects one in five people and is a major cause of lost working days. Around 12 million people in the UK and some 36 million Americans experience symptoms at some time in their lives. And for 10–15 per cent, the symptoms will be sufficiently troublesome to prompt them to seek medical help.

Over half of all people attending gastroenterology out-patient clinics have IBS. Indeed, the condition is the most common reason to be referred to such a clinic. However, an estimated three-quarters of IBS sufferers never see a doctor. And many of those who do seek medical advice, feel that they get frustratingly little help.

The cause of IBS remains a mystery and doctors are often as baffled as sufferers by the diversity of symptoms and the difficulty of finding an effective treatment. The good news is that with all the research today, doctors are beginning to understand more about the condition.

Most IBS sufferers know that what they eat can provoke or alleviate symptoms and, increasingly, research is beginning to pinpoint exactly which foods may help and which may make symptoms worse. Encouragingly, the diet recommended for people with IBS is the very same one that is generally believed to be vital for a long, healthy life – that is a diet rich in fresh fruits and vegetables, oily fish, nuts, seeds and cereals.

Of course IBS is not caused by, nor can it be prevented by, any single factor, and even diet, vital though it can be, is not the whole story. This book aims to help you understand the many different aspects of irritable bowel syndrome.

It begins by looking at the digestive system and how it works, and explains how in people who suffer from IBS the digestive system may work differently. It also examines some of the fascinating theories that are now emerging about the causes of IBS and, in particular, some of the intriguing links between the brain and the gut.

In Chapter 2 you will learn about all the potential factors that can trigger IBS symptoms and how you can begin to control them. This chapter also contains tips on how to manage IBS at work, rest and play.

Chapter 3 takes a look at the orthodox medical approach and all the tests your doctor might do to diagnose IBS, in addition to treatments that may be prescribed or are available over the counter.

IBS is a difficult condition to treat and even doctors agree that the treatments currently on offer only have limited success. Perhaps for this reason a great many people with IBS consult complementary therapists. Chapter 4 contains details of some of the complementary therapies that may be most useful in treating IBS, outlining what you can expect from a therapist, how he or she may help and some of the exciting new research into these therapies.

Chapter 5 takes an extensive look at the role of food in IBS, showing you how you can eat better and control your symptoms, as well as looking at the latest thinking about fibre and other food factors.

The book concludes with two chapters of recipes designed to help you to eat more healthily and control your symptoms. Chapter 6 is devoted to recipes for people who are sensitive to certain types of food, while Chapter 7 contains a host of delicious, nutritious dishes that can help improve your overall diet and rekindle your enjoyment of food.

The aim of this book is to increase your knowledge of how you can take control of irritable bowel syndrome. Whether you have IBS yourself or are close to someone with it, you will find a host of useful information that will enable you to stay healthy and feel better.

# 1 Irritable bowel syndrome explained

Virtually everyone experiences some symptoms of irritable bowel – abdominal pain, bloating, constipation and diarrhoea – at one time or another. What distinguishes people with IBS from other people is that these symptoms occur together and last over a period of time.

For some sufferers the symptoms of IBS constitute little more than an occasional nuisance. However, others are affected more severely and an unfortunate few are crippled by stomach cramps, constipation or diarrhoea, necessitating constant trips to the lavatory.

Understanding the possible causes and triggers can enable you to control symptoms and take charge so that IBS does not rule your life. This chapter explains what IBS is and how it relates to your digestive system. It details the symptoms, and explores the theories as to their causes. Understanding the nature of your condition can help put you on the road to an IBS-free life, or at the very least help reduce your symptoms.

# Defining IBS

Irritable bowel syndrome is not a disease as such, but a condition or disorder. The term 'syndrome' refers to a fixed pattern of symptoms that occur together. These symptoms are all linked to a particular disorder. In IBS these symptoms include abdominal pain, changes in bowel habit, changes in stools and a swollen abdomen.

IBS is a chronic condition, one that is present over a long period of time, although attacks can be acute, that is symptoms may flare up rapidly.

Over the years many different names have been used to describe IBS. They include colitis, mucous colitis, spastic colon, spastic bowel, nervous colon and irritable colon. Not only are these terms outdated but they can also be extremely misleading, suggesting a clear-cut physical cause such as inflammation (colitis means, literally, inflammation of the colon), or fostering the equally inaccurate idea that IBS is all in the mind.

# Functional bowel disorders

IBS is the most common of a number of conditions described by doctors as functional bowel disorders. This term indicates cases where the way the bowel works or functions has altered rather than detectable changes in the bowel with an obvious physical cause such as inflammation, faulty development or a chemical imbalance.

An irritable bowel looks perfectly normal and healthy, both to the naked eye and when examined under a microscope.

Unfortunately, until fairly recently, this has sometimes led to IBS being dismissed as psychosomatic and to sufferers being labelled as neurotic. As with many illnesses there is a mind-body connection in IBS, but that does not mean that your symptoms are imaginary. Thankfully, as more and more is discovered about IBS and its causes, these unhelpful labels are being abandoned.

# Who gets IBS?

IBS can affect anyone at any age, but most often the symptoms develop between the ages of 15 and 40. It is rare for IBS to develop for the first time after the age of 50, although symptoms can of course persist beyond this age.

Although IBS affects men and women in equal numbers, women are three times more likely to seek help from their doctor and symptoms are often worse before and during the first few days of a period.

IBS has been diagnosed all over the world and is as common in China, India, Japan and South America as it is in the West, although some experts have suggested that it is less common in South East Asia and Africa. In the developing world, symptoms seem to be more common in people living in towns and cities than those living in rural areas.

# True or false?
## IBS is all in the mind

False. To the extent that IBS is not due to anatomical or structural defects, and tests come back normal, it is not a physical disease.

However, as with many conditions, symptoms can be exacerbated by stress and anxiety. This does not mean that they are all in the mind. Recent research suggests that the messenger chemicals in the gut that communicate with the brain play a significant part, so you could equally well claim that IBS is 'all in the gut'.

## IBS is caused by food allergy

True and false. Most studies do not indicate that IBS is caused by food allergy proper, in the sense that the body's immune system over-reacts. However, research does show that a proportion of people who suffer from IBS may be sensitive to certain foods.

## You can catch IBS

False. IBS is not transmissible by viruses or bacteria. On the other hand, it can be triggered by a bout of gastroenteritis (for example, food poisoning or holiday tummy) and research suggests that it can also be a result of excessive growth of normal bacteria in the gut.

## IBS runs in families

True and false. IBS is not generally considered to be hereditary. However, because it is extremely common, if you do have IBS you may find that other members of your family may have similar symptoms. In addition to this, researchers are looking at whether an inherited fault in the autonomic nervous system, which controls automatic actions such as heart rate, breathing and bowel contractions, may be a causal factor in some people.

## IBS is caused by inflammation

False. Unlike organic bowel diseases, such as ulcerative colitis and Crohn's disease, IBS is not caused by inflammation, although where food sensitivity is involved there may be an inflammatory component.

## IBS can cause serious digestive disease

False. IBS does not cause other gastrointestinal diseases and nor is it caused by ulcers, gallstones, cancer or other more serious digestive diseases.

# Symptoms of IBS

The symptoms of IBS can vary, both from person to person and from time to time. If you suspect that you suffer from IBS, you should be on the look out for a pattern of continuous or recurrent symptoms persisting over a period of at least three months. These include:

## Abdominal pain or discomfort

Pain – usually intermittent – is felt anywhere in the abdomen but often low down on the left-hand side. Pain may be worse if you are constipated and can be relieved when you open your bowels or break wind. Women often find abdominal discomfort is worse before or during a period.

## Feeling full or bloated/abdominal distension

You feel uncomfortably full and your waistband digs in. Your abdomen may feel tender to touch. Often bloating gets worse as the day goes on. This may be linked to a rumbling stomach and flatulence.

## Changed bowel habits

Some people with IBS have painful loose stools or diarrhoea, some have painful hard stools or constipation, others alternate between the two. IBS can cause bowel motions to become more or less frequent and may be associated with a desperate need to empty the bowels.

## A sensation of incomplete emptying

In IBS there is often the feeling that there is more stool to be passed, even immediately after having a bowel motion. This can lead to ineffective straining, medically known as tenesmus. It may also bring on a sharp pain in the anus known as proctalgia fugax.

## Mucus in the stool

In IBS it is possible that the mucus glands in the walls of the bowels may become overactive due to prolonged contact with slow-moving motions. This can result in the passage of hard, pellet-like stools that are covered in mucus. You may also pass just mucus.

# How severe is IBS?

The symptoms of IBS can be mild and cause only occasional problems, for example, you may experience a bout of stomach ache before you open your bowels or a desperate urge to go first thing in the morning.

At the other end of the scale, some sufferers are totally incapacitated by their symptoms. Although the symptoms may be severe, IBS is not severe in the sense that it is progressive or life threatening.

## Other symptoms associated with IBS

Many people with IBS have other symptoms affecting other parts of the body as well as the bowel.

**Feeling sick and feeling full**  Nausea (feeling sick) is a common feature of IBS, although actual vomiting is fairly rare. Sufferers also complain of feeling uncomfortably full after eating only a small quantity of food, a phenomenon doctors call early satiety.

**Irritable bladder**  Some people with irritable bowel also seem to have an over-reactive bladder. Symptoms of an irritable bladder include frequency (needing to pass urine more often), urgency (feeling a desperate urge to pass urine), nocturia (needing to go to the toilet during the night) and a feeling of incomplete emptying.

**Migraine and tension headaches**  Some sufferers of IBS appear to be more prone to migraine and tension headaches.

**Painful sex and periods**  Women may experience painful intercourse (dyspareunia) and periods (dysmenorrhea).

**Tiredness, lethargy, chronic fatigue**  Some people with IBS also experience feelings of being tired all the time.

**Heartburn**  Chest pain caused by the reflux of stomach acids is often associated with heartburn, although it has many causes.

**Fibromyalgia**  Fibromyalgia sufferers are plagued by muscular aches and pains and stiffness, with tenderness of specific trigger points. It is often accompanied by fatigue and tiredness and other symptoms. In the past few years doctors have increasingly observed that people with fibromyalgia are likely to have symptoms of IBS.

**Psychological symptoms**  IBS may be associated with anxiety, frustration or depression.

**Asthma** IBS sufferers are more likely to develop asthma, a condition which is caused by oversensitivity of the airways (bronchial hyperactivity).

The presence of these non-intestinal symptoms has led some doctors to surmise that IBS might be part of a more generalized problem affecting smooth muscle tissue (a specialized muscle tissue found in all the parts of the body where the above symptoms occur) and not just a condition of the gastrointestinal tract or the abdominal organs.

## The power of mind over body

Some doctors – mainly psychiatrists – believe IBS to be due to 'somatization', whereby emotional stress, anxiety and depression are expressed in physical symptoms. Not surprisingly, some people with IBS feel annoyed by this definition because it infers that their symptoms are not real. In fact, doctors who specialize in somatization disorders stress that this is not the case. The symptoms are real enough, they assert, but are not due to physical disease.

# The digestive system

A knowledge of how the bowel normally works can help you better understand what goes wrong in IBS. The term 'bowel' refers to the colon, part of the large intestine or gut, which in turn is part of the digestive or gastrointestinal system.

A healthy gastrointestinal system is vital for life. It is here that everything we eat and drink is broken down and converted into the raw materials our cells need to fuel and nourish our bodies, from the day we are born until the moment we die.

# The digestive tract

The digestive tract, also known as the gastrointestinal tract or alimentary canal, is a muscular tube, about 9 m (30 ft) long, that winds through your body from your mouth to your anus (back passage). It operates as a processing plant, where food is ingested and broken down into nutrients. The nutrients are absorbed into the bloodstream and any indigestible waste is expelled from the body. Food takes from 24 to 72 hours to pass through the system.

The digestive tract comprises the mouth, the pharynx, the oesophagus, the stomach, the small intestine and the large intestine. Other organs involved in the process of digestion include the teeth, tongue and gallbladder. The salivary glands, the liver and the pancreas secrete the enzymes needed to break down food.

# The digestive process

When you eat a meal, the food is chewed, mixed, moulded and moistened with saliva. This begins the process of chemical breakdown.

The softened ball of food (bolus) is swallowed and propelled into the pharynx, a muscle-lined cavity at the back of the throat. From here it is propelled by a series of wave-like contractions into the oesophagus, or gullet.

## The oesophagus

The oesophagus – an elastic tube about 25 cm (10 in) long – consists of four layers: a lining of mucus membrane which enables food to slide down, a submucosal layer, a thick layer of muscle and an outer protective coat.

## WHAT HAPPENS TO THE FOOD WE EAT?

Digestion is a complex process that demands the synchronization of a whole range of activities and processes. Broadly speaking, digestion involves two key processes. These are:

1 Mechanical digestion, in which your body prepares the food for chemical digestion by enzymes. Mechanical digestion includes chewing, mixing food with saliva and churning food in the stomach.

2 Chemical digestion, in which food molecules are broken down by enzymes so that they can be absorbed into the bloodstream. The process begins in your mouth and is completed in the small intestine.

In reality, mechanical and chemical digestion cannot be separated so clearly.

## The stomach

From the oesophagus, food passes into the stomach, a J-shaped muscular sac approximately 25 cm (10 in) long, which acts as a reservoir for food and converts it into a creamy paste called chyme. When empty, your stomach has a volume of around 50 ml (2 fl oz), but it can expand to hold up to 4 litres (just under a gallon).

In the stomach, food is churned, mixed, pummelled and broken down into even smaller fragments. Gastric juices, acids and enzymes – secreted by the gastric glands – break the food down into its component parts of proteins, starches, fats and sugars over a period of several hours.

# The small intestine

The chyme passes from the stomach into the small intestine, where virtually all digestion and absorption of nutrients takes place. In the first part of the small intestine, the duodenum, acidic stomach contents are neutralized by a number of different secretions.

Food then passes into the next part of the small intestine, the jejunum – yet another tube – the interior of which consists of a series of circular folds. These allow liquified food and nutrients to be absorbed into the bloodstream. Some of the fatty components of food are absorbed into the lymphatic system here. What remains of the chyme passes into the final part of the small intestine, the ileum, a 3.5 m (12 ft) long tube where more nutrients are absorbed.

# The large intestine

The solid products remaining after food has been absorbed in the small intestine now enter the large intestine, also known as the hind gut or large bowel. The first part of the large intestine is the colon, another tube, measuring about 1.3 m (4¼ ft).

The colon's job is to move waste matter to the anus by means of waves of muscular contractions (peristalsis), and to absorb salts and water to create a solid stool. Around 2.4 litres (4¼ pints) of liquid matter enter the colon from the small intestine each day. Most of the time the colon barely moves a muscle. However, following a meal, it contracts at points along its length. Contractions typically occur 10 cm (4 in) apart at 10-minute intervals. This helps slow down the flow of waste and keeps it in contact with the bowel wall so that water can be absorbed. Bacterial fermentation in the bowel helps break down the undigested food and processes the undigested fibre, which can take several days.

The stool then passes through the colon to the rectum, yet another muscular tube, where it is stored until you open your bowels. The rectum is lined with a membrane known as the epithelium. This contains mucus glands which lubricate the stool and make it easier to pass. The final part of the digestive tract is the anus or anal canal, the opening through which the solid waste, now known as faeces, is expelled. Faeces are normally made up of 75 per cent water and 25 per cent solids.

# What goes wrong in IBS?

While the exact causes of IBS remain a mystery, there are some intriguing clues. Scientists have identified several ways in which the gut does not act normally in people with IBS. Firstly, the muscular activity, or motility, of the gut may be altered in people with IBS. Secondly, it is possible that people with IBS may have a lowered sensation threshold for pain or pressure, although this is by no means a general rule. Thirdly, there may be disturbances in the way the brain and gut communicate with each other.

## Changes in motility

The term 'motility' refers to the muscular activity of the gut. Motility is controlled by messages from nerves, hormones and the electrical activity of the colon muscle, which acts rather like a pacemaker in the heart.

Normally when you eat, the presence of food stimulates the muscles of the gastrointestinal tract to contract and relax rhythmically, to propel food through the system.

Research suggests that this process is disordered in people with IBS. This means that instead of food being propelled smoothly along the digestive tract, contractions either speed up, causing diarrhoea, or slow down, causing constipation.

In one famous piece of research carried out at the John Hopkins University in the USA, researchers found that healthy people have between six and eight peristaltic contractions in the colon per day, whereas people with IBS have as few as none or as many as 25, depending on whether constipation or diarrhoea is dominant.

Another interesting finding is that in IBS sufferers the colon tends to go into spasm after only mild stimulation. Therefore, normal stimuli, such as a meal or wind in the bowel, cause the colon to contract more strongly and more painfully.

Doctors have also looked at differences in small bowel (small intestine) activity and found that people with IBS are prone to short bursts of intense activity followed by long intervals of rest, called clustered contractions. Some of these seem to coincide with bouts of abdominal pain.

Researchers have also studied transit time, the time a stool takes to pass through the gut. Where diarrhoea is a dominant symptom, transit time is much faster than in healthy volunteers. Unfortunately, however, not all studies find clear-cut differences between healthy people and people with IBS, so abnormal motility is clearly not the whole story.

## Altered sensation

Doctors have been arguing for years about whether people with IBS sense abnormal movements of the gut normally or whether they sense normal movements of the gut abnormally.

Research suggests that in some people with IBS the nerves in the gastrointestinal tract respond differently to stimuli such as food in the gut. More precisely, it is thought that they have a lower sensation threshold for pressure or pain. This means that even normal contractions of the bowel induce pain.

This has been demonstrated in studies where a balloon has been blown up in the rectum to mimic what happens when wind or waste matter passes through the gut. For example, in a series of studies, again performed at John Hopkins University in the USA, scientists found that people without IBS reported moderate pain when the balloon's volume reached about 160 ml (5½ fl oz). However, people with IBS experienced pain at just 60 ml (2½ fl oz).

This increased sensitivity means that a harmless bubble of wind, which most people would barely notice, can cause acute discomfort or pain in IBS sufferers. Unfortunately, as with virtually everything to do with IBS, not all studies agree with each other. In fact, some studies have shown that IBS sufferers are less sensitive to pain than others. So this is not the whole story either.

## Bacterial overgrowth

Recent research suggests that IBS may be caused by the presence of too many of the normal bacteria that inhabit the small intestine. Bacterial overgrowth, as this is called, is linked to typical IBS symptoms such as bloating, abdominal cramps and diarrhoea.

Bacteria cause fermentation in the bowel, a by-product of which is the gas hydrogen. In a research project reported in the *American Journal of Gastroenterology*, over three-quarters of IBS patients tested with a breath test had higher than normal levels of hydrogen, suggesting bacterial overgrowth. Forty-seven of these patients were then treated with antibiotics. After treatment, more than half of them experienced an improvement in their IBS symptoms.

Admittedly, the number of people studied was only small – just 157 patients. However, if bacterial overgrowth does prove a significant factor even in a few people, it could lead to a revolution in treatment.

## Irritable bowel or irritable body?

Some scientists suggest that the bodies of people with IBS are generally more sensitive to stimuli than those of others, in much the same way that some people have sensitive skin which is more prone to sunburn. Support for this theory comes from the fact that people with IBS are more likely to experience nausea and feel full after eating only a small amount of food. And, as we've seen, they are also more likely to have other non-intestinal symptoms.

A common factor that unites all these diverse symptoms (see pages 17–18) is the presence of smooth muscle tissue in the parts of the body affected. Smooth muscle tissue is a specialized type of muscle which can contract in all directions simultaneously and is not under voluntary control. It usually constitutes the walls of tube-like structures such as the digestive tract, the urinary tract, the arteries and the vagina. This has led some experts to surmise that in some people the body's control of smooth muscle function is disrupted.

One supporter of this theory is UK-based gastroenterologist Professor Michael Farthing, who wrote in the *British Medical*

*Journal*, 'instead of merely an irritable bowel, there might also be an irritable oesophagus, an irritable stomach, an irritable bladder and irritable vagina, and possibly irritable bronchi – or simply an irritable body.'

## The brain-gut connection

Some of the most exciting research over the past few years has been in a new field of science called neuro-gastroenterology, which is an area that is concerned with the links between the brain and the gut.

As the term 'gut reaction' might suggest, there are strong connections between our emotions and our guts. There are few of us who haven't experienced a churning stomach before an important event; the stress of an impending exam or interview can make us feel quite literally sick with nerves and rob us of appetite. Studies have shown that anger, loud music or being woken suddenly from sleep can all increase gut motility, while feeling calm decreases it. At the same time, the movement of the gut as it digests can affect our emotional state. Just think how a bout of indigestion can make you feel thoroughly miserable and bad tempered.

In recent years, scientists have discovered that our guts have their own nervous system, complete with the very same chemicals found in the brain and spinal cord. This second brain, as it is often known, can function both on its own and can also communicate with our main brain by means of messenger chemicals.

In fact, the whole lining of the gut is teeming with these messenger chemicals and is also rich in receptors (places where messenger chemicals bind to cells rather like a key fitting into a lock). These chemicals help to control what we feel and how we perceive. They are in constant communication both with the brain and central nervous system and with other parts of the gastrointestinal system.

One of the chemicals that has been much studied over the past few years is serotonin (5HT), sometimes known as the happiness hormone, which helps to control mood and appetite. A lack of serotonin has been found to be a major factor in depression and other mood disorders.

These exciting findings are paving the way for the development of new drugs and treatments, which act not simply to quell symptoms, as most existing ones do, but work directly on the brain to correct imbalances of chemicals and calm the gut.

## Mood and personality

The new knowledge about the connections between the brain and the gut may eventually shed some light on the important role that mood and personality can play in IBS. There is no doubt that a negative mood can exacerbate the symptoms of IBS – as of course it can any illness. However, although many studies have looked into this, as with so many aspects of this puzzling condition they seem to raise as many questions as they answer.

In some studies, IBS sufferers have been found to be more anxious and more than usually concerned about their health. And in an Australian study carried out in 2001, researchers looking at patients with IBS and unexplained abdominal pain found that they shared distinct personality traits. These patients reported feeling less cared for by those close to them, were less assertive or over-aggressive in getting their needs met and perceived themselves to be less in control of their lives than others.

Whether this amounts to an IBS personality, however, remains debatable. For a start, not everyone with IBS is anxious. Furthermore, many people with the condition have had perfectly well-behaved bowels until a bout of holiday tummy or food poisoning unsettled their gut.

So what are we to conclude? It could be that mood disturbance or an anxious personality leads to abdominal pain and discomfort. But, equally, it could be that IBS leads to a greater awareness of mild symptoms that previously went unnoticed. It could also be that nagging abdominal symptoms trigger anxiety and insecurity. The truth is no one really knows.

To sum up, no one as yet knows what causes IBS and it seems likely that there are different causes in different people and in different types of IBS. Only time will tell.

## In the genes?

Although IBS is not thought to be inherited in the strict sense, genes may be involved. Some research suggests that IBS symptoms may be associated with a fault in the autonomic nervous system (the system that controls all the body's day-to-day functions, such as breathing and heart rate), which makes the gut more prone to react to sudden fluctuations in blood circulation to the abdomen. And in one study carried out in the USA, researchers found that a faulty gene, involved in panic attacks and anxiety, was present in a group of women with IBS. The number studied was too small to draw any definitive conclusions. However, it is a promising line of enquiry and, with the explosion of gene research currently taking place, over the next few years there may be more definite evidence of genetic links which could help doctors tailor treatments more effectively to individual sufferers.

# 2 Managing IBS

The severity of IBS varies greatly from person to person and it seems almost certain that some of this is due to lifestyle. Some IBS sufferers are conscious that symptoms are most marked during times of stress and anxiety. However, this is by no means always the case. In fact, in many people, symptoms seem to strike completely out of the blue with no apparent cause. In some instances, the symptoms go away of their own accord, leaving the sufferer with long symptom-free periods.

In many cases it may be possible to avoid or even avert flare-ups of symptoms by identifying potential triggers and avoiding them where possible. Learning all the possible triggers of your irritable bowel can be a time-consuming exercise. However, it is one that is extremely worthwhile because it can help you to gain a sense of control.

Over the years, gastrointestinal experts have identified certain factors that are know to commonly spark off IBS symptoms. Many experts now believe that the bodies of people with IBS are particularly sensitive to stimulation either from within or outside their bodies.

## What's normal?

Bowel function varies greatly from one individual to another. There are simply no rules. It is perfectly within the bounds of normal experience to empty your bowels between anything from three times a day to three times a week. A normal stool is passed without cramping or pain, is formed but not hard and contains no blood.

## Identifying patterns

The first step is to identify what sparks off your symptoms. Becoming aware of your own personal trigger factors and doing what you can to eliminate or control them can help you reduce the number of attacks or the severity of symptoms.

We are all unique individuals, so you may find that the factors which spark off your symptoms are different to those that affect other people. Having said that however, there do appear to be certain common triggers that affect many people with IBS.

One point to bear in mind is that some triggers may affect you more than others. Another is that you may find that triggers vary at different times. For example, if you are a woman you may find that certain factors are especially likely to trigger symptoms around the time of your period. Some people with IBS find that stress and anxiety aggravate symptoms, yet others don't – keep an open mind, be honest and concentrate on finding out what factors are important for you rather than simply believing everything the 'experts' say.

# Trigger diaries

The easiest way to pinpoint your own personal IBS triggers is to keep a diary of your symptoms together with a note detailing associated factors. After a few weeks you will probably begin to notice patterns emerging which can help you identify things that set off your symptoms. If you decide to seek medical help, you can show the diary to your doctor to enable him or her to reach a more accurate diagnosis.

You may already have a fair idea of some of the factors that trigger your symptoms. However, keeping a diary will enable you to pinpoint those which are most significant and whether just one or several are needed before you develop symptoms.

## Avoiding common triggers

There are many possible IBS triggers, including insufficient dietary fibre, food intolerance, infections, certain drugs, stress, menstruation and smoking. Although each person is different, it is extremely likely that one or more of these triggers will affect you.

Some triggers are relatively simple to avoid. For example, if certain foods cause problems, you can steer clear of them. Others may be more difficult to control, for example if your symptoms are made worse by stress, travelling or, if you are a woman, by menstruation. Nonetheless, to be forewarned is to be forearmed and with a bit of planning it is often possible to anticipate and minimize the effects of many triggers.

## How to keep a trigger diary

Keeping a trigger diary is extremely simple. You can either use your ordinary diary if it has space or, alternatively, you might like to buy a special diary or notebook for the purpose. Keep this in a handy place and whenever you experience symptoms record the following information:

1 Date and time of symptoms
2 Specific symptoms, such as diarrhoea, constipation, bloating, abdominal pain. Include non-bowel symptoms too, such as urinary problems, headache, asthma
3 Severity of symptoms – mild, moderate, severe or very severe. Alternatively, you could record these on a scale of one to five
4 How your symptoms progressed, what eased them (for example opening your bowels) and what made them worse
5 Any action you took (including any medication) and whether it had any effect
6 How long symptoms lasted

In the same notebook or diary, or on a separate sheet of paper, record potential triggers. Include details of:

❑ Your diet: what you ate and drank
❑ Activities and exercise or lack of activity
❑ Details of any journeys or travel
❑ Work or social events and activities
❑ Any medications you took, including over-the-counter, natural or herbal remedies
❑ If you are a woman, make a note of the dates of your menstrual periods and any symptoms associated with premenstrual syndrome, pregnancy or the menopause

# Food and drinks

Because IBS is a disorder of the digestive system, many experts believe that what you eat and drink is crucial. That's not to say that diet causes IBS, but that it can be one of the key triggers. There is no single food or type of food that sparks symptoms in everyone who suffers from IBS, but there are certain foods that are frequently implicated. You can find details in Chapter 5, pages 110–113.

Despite the evidence of a food connection, experts are still not entirely sure why food triggers symptoms of IBS. Some people may have a food sensitivity, although many doctors dismiss this idea.

More controversial still is the idea, supported mainly by complementary and alternative practitioners, that candidiasis, a chronic condition caused by the yeast *Candida albicans*, may be involved (see page 114).

Where constipation is a dominant symptom, lack of fibre may be a factor, although some people with IBS find that too much fibre actually triggers symptoms.

## Take action

❑ You may be able to bring your symptoms under control by watching what you eat and drink.

❑ In order to be effective this needs to be done in a systematic way so that you can monitor the precise effects of different foods.

❑ In all but the simplest cases this is best done under the supervision of a doctor, dietician or nutritional therapist. You'll find further details and a lot more about how to adjust your diet in Chapter 5, pages 93–119.

# Smoking

Many people with IBS find that exposure to smoke, even second-hand smoke, worsens symptoms. However, while most of us know the harmful effects smoking has on the heart and lungs, few are aware of the devastation it can wreak on the digestive system.

When you inhale, smoke enters the stomach and intestines, not just the lungs. Nicotine stimulates the adrenal glands, triggering a stress response. It also has a direct effect on the nerves that control the bowel wall and affect its activity, leading to the familiar symptoms of bloating, abdominal pain, wind and stomach rumbling.

Smoking is also associated with other digestive conditions, namely acid reflux, heartburn, peptic ulcer and Crohn's disease. It can also change the way your liver handles drugs and alcohol.

## Take action

❑ In the light of the above, it really is worth trying to quit, even if you have tried before. The most effective way to change an unhealthy habit is to think of it as a journey, involving several milestones.

❑ Before you even start, make a list of everything you will gain from quitting smoking, including everything from better health to more money.

❑ Enlist the support of family and friends by telling them of your intention to stop. Having a quitting companion can help strengthen your resolve. If your partner or someone in your household smokes, he or she could be the ideal person, because passive smoking can affect your irritable bowel. However, if he or she doesn't want to quit, don't use this as an excuse for not doing anything.

❑ Joining a stop-smoking group can help motivate you, especially if you are the sort of person who does well in a class or group situation.

❑ If you prefer to go it alone, check out books, tapes, videos and the Internet. There's plenty of help out there if you look for it.

❑ One thing that can help is to become aware of your personal smoking cues, the things you associate with lighting up. For example, you may always light up after supper or have a cigarette at 11am with a cup of coffee. An important part of quitting is to break these habits, for example by going for a run after supper or phoning a friend, or having a (healthy) snack instead of a cigarette with a mug of herbal tea at 11am – treat yourself to a piece of exotic fruit and really savour it.

❑ Some people find hypnotherapy or acupuncture helpful (see Chapter 4, pages 74–76 and 89). Your doctor can also be a great source of help and can prescribe nicotine replacement therapy – patches, gums or sprays – or other stop-smoking aids.

## Female hormones

IBS symptoms such as bloating, constipation, diarrhoea and abdominal pain are common just before and during the first few days of menstruation. A common pattern is to be bloated and constipated premenstrually, and have abdominal cramps and diarrhoea at the onset of menstruation. Experts recognize that many medical problems, such as headaches and migraine, asthma and chronic fatigue, are worse before a period, a phenomenon known as menstrual magnification. No one knows exactly why this happens, but female hormones are known to affect the gut, and other chemicals linked to the menstrual cycle may also be involved.

One of the prime culprits may be the female sex hormone progesterone, which is dominant during the second half of the menstrual cycle and helps prepare your body for a potential pregnancy. Among its effects are the relaxation of smooth muscle tissue throughout the body. In the gut this leads to slower bowel transit time and constipation.

Also possibly involved are the chemicals known as prostaglandins, hormone-like substances produced in all the body's cells. One of the jobs of prostaglandins, which is relevant both to IBS and PMS, is that they help to control inflammatory reactions.

One particular group of prostaglandins has been associated with diarrhoea during menstruation and has also been linked to causing contractions of the uterus and the smooth muscle tissue of the intestine. This could be a possible explanation for why some women with IBS also complain of periods that are painful and uncomfortable.

Experts have identified several links between bowel and gynaecological problems. For example, one in ten women who have a hysterectomy subsequently develop IBS symptoms, although the reason is not clear and in other women symptoms actually abate after the operation. Constipation can often be a problem during pregnancy too, when progesterone levels act to relax smooth muscle tissue in order to prepare the body for birth.

IBS may also co-exist with and worsen menopausal symptoms, although it is not a symptom of the menopause as such. If you are taking HRT to control menopausal symptoms, the hormones used may affect the activity of the bowel.

## Take action

❑ Being aware of the effect hormonal changes have on your symptoms can enable you to begin to control them. As we have already discussed, keeping a symptom diary can help, as can watching your diet (see Chapter 5, pages 93–113).

❑ You might consider taking evening primrose oil and increasing your consumption of oily fish. The essential fatty acids found in these help to balance prostaglandin levels and also may reduce pain and inflammation and aid digestion.

**Note:** if you have any form of epilepsy, you shouldn't take evening primrose oil without the advice of your doctor or qualified nutritionist. If you have blood disorders or bleeding problems, fish oils should only be taken under medical supervision.

❑ Learning how to manage stress (see pages 42–45) is another important step, since stress hormones, like adrenalin and the brain chemical noradrenalin, are implicated in both IBS and PMS.

❑ The herb *Agnus castus*, which is known to help balance hormones, has been found to be useful in treating IBS symptoms in women. For more details on herbal treatments see Chapter 4, pages 82–84 and 89–92. For further information on dealing with PMS see our companion book *Food Solutions: PMS*.

# Drugs and medicines

A large number of prescribed and over-the-counter drugs can affect the way the bowels work. Analgesic (pain killing) medications, such as aspirin, and non-steroidal anti-inflammatory drugs (NSAIDs), like ibuprofen, are particular culprits in causing diarrhoea and abdominal discomfort. Other offending medications include certain types of laxatives which can cause diarrhoea, anti-depressants of the tricyclic group which can cause constipation, iron tablets which can cause constipation, codeine which can also cause constipation, and caffeine, found in some pain killers, which can cause diarrhoea. Many IBS sufferers report that their problems developed after a course of antibiotics (although see Chapter 1, pages 24–25 for the role antibiotics can play in curing some people of the symptoms of IBS). Antibiotics work by killing harmful bacteria. However, in the process they can also wipe out normal good bacteria that live in the bowel and help with digestion.

## Take action

❑ Try to avoid all medications unless they are strictly necessary.

❑ When prescribed a drug or buying one over the counter in the pharmacy, always tell the doctor or pharmacist that you have IBS and read the packet insert carefully to check for additives and whether indigestion or bowel problems are potential side effects.

❑ If you are prescribed antibiotics, try eating lots of live yogurt or taking an acidophilus supplement to help recolonize your gut with good bacteria. Don't ever stop taking a prescribed drug without consulting your doctor.

# Sleep and sleep patterns

A number of studies are beginning to look at the part sleeping habits may play in triggering IBS symptoms. Several have shown an alteration in bowel function during sleep in sufferers; others have found that people with IBS have more rapid eye movement (REM) sleep – a type of sleep associated with dreaming. Another study identified links between the severity of morning IBS symptoms and a poor night's sleep. It is not entirely clear what the significance of these studies is. However, if you detect a link between your symptoms and the quality of your sleep, it can do no harm to practise good sleep hygiene, as outlined below.

## Take action

- ❑ Try to go to bed at the same time every night, even at weekends.
- ❑ Wind down slowly during the evening and avoid stimulating television programmes, videos, listening to loud music or other activities before turning in.
- ❑ Avoid heavy meals, especially fatty meals, before bedtime, and avoid alcohol as this can make you feel sleepy initially but wake you up later on and increases the amount of REM sleep.
- ❑ A mug of camomile tea or a warm milky drink, if you can tolerate milk, before you go to bed will help relax you.
- ❑ Have a warm bath or shower before bed.
- ❑ Make sure your bedroom is a comfortable temperature: not too warm or too cold.
- ❑ Your bedroom should be a haven you use just for sleeping. Clear out the television, books and newspapers, and never take work to bed with you.

# Stress and tension

The general consensus is that stress doesn't cause IBS as such. Having said that, physical and emotional tension affects virtually everyone's digestive system. And in IBS sufferers the gut may be particularly prone to react to stress. Research reported at a major conference on gastrointestinal disorders in 2001, for example, showed that when IBS sufferers who had diarrhoea as a dominant symptom were subjected to stress, they exhibited a stronger emotional response and their perceptions of discomfort were stronger than those experienced by a control group.

## Stressful life events

Life events are any events that cause a major change in your social and personal circumstances – either positive or negative. The types of life events reported by people with IBS vary from person to person. They can include, in no particular order:

❑ Loss of a parent or partner by death, divorce or separation

❑ Injury or illness

❑ Loss of a job or moving to a new job

❑ Moving house

❑ Retirement

❑ Changes in your daily routine, such as changed working hours or conditions

❑ Health problems

❑ Pregnancy and/or the arrival of a new baby

❑ Changes in your relationship with your partner, such as arguments or sexual difficulties

❑ Trouble with relatives or friends

❑ Changes in eating or sleeping habits

❑ Going on holiday or time off work
❑ Older children leaving home

## So what exactly is stress and how does It act on your bowels?

Quite simply, it is your body's reaction to challenge. Whenever you are faced with a new situation, a complex biochemical chain reaction occurs in your body, which is known as the stress response.

Stress hormones, such as adrenalin and the brain chemical noradrenalin, are released at times of stress, and these hormones cause a rise in blood pressure, heart rate, oxygen intake and blood flow to the muscles.

Crucially for IBS sufferers, stress hormones also act on the digestive system, causing the bowel to contract more rapidly to help us rid ourselves of food that might slow us down if we had to fight or flee. For our ancestors, this fight or flight reaction could quite literally make the difference between life and death and, even today, in certain situations it can still help us to cope with difficult or unusual circumstances. However, for the IBS sufferer it can cause internal havoc.

## Take action

Obviously you can't eradicate stress completely. Nor would you wish to – too little stress leads to boredom, apathy and lack of motivation. However, you can learn to anticipate and manage it.

❑ Keep a record (another use for that diary) of people and things that make you feel stressed, to help you develop tactics to deal with them and to plan in advance. For example, if you have a stressful event such as a holiday or an exam coming up, visualizing it in detail and planning to deal with it calmly can help avoid panic – and intestinal hurry.

❑ Time management is another vital skill and there are many books and other resources you can use to learn it.

❑ Learn to be assertive and say 'No' without feeling guilty – remember IBS sufferers may be less assertive in their relationships. Learning to deal appropriately with anger can also help.

❑ Of course, by their very nature, not all stressful events can be anticipated. In this case, developing a battery of techniques for helping you to relax is essential.

## Relaxation techniques

There are various types of relaxation technique. One method involves alternately tensing and relaxing each group of muscles in turn from your toes to your head. By the time you have finished, your body should be completely relaxed. Another method involves concentrating on your breathing.

Here's a simple, yoga-based breathing technique you can practise anywhere:

1 Sit comfortably or lie down if possible, loosen your waistband if it is tight and remove other tight clothing. Pull the blind or curtains if you find it helpful.

2 Slowly become aware of your breathing and try to make the out-breath the same length as the in-breath.

3 Gradually deepen your breathing so that as you breathe in your stomach swells, then your ribcage, then your chest. As you breathe out, let your stomach fall, then your ribcage, then your chest.

**4** Now lengthen each breath to a count of nine seconds. Mentally count in and out: stomach, two, three, ribcage, five, six, chest, eight, nine. Stomach, two, three, ribcage, five, six, chest, eight, nine.

**5** Extend this to 12 seconds, then let your breathing return to normal, natural breathing and just sit or lie there for a while feeling deeply relaxed.

# Exercise and exertion

Regular moderate activity helps stimulate circulation, lowers blood pressure, tones your muscles and boosts immunity. What is less often mentioned is that it can also aid digestion. Exercise helps regulate the peristaltic waves that propel food through your digestive tract, and so it can help alleviate constipation. Secondly, by enhancing your metabolism, it can increase your uptake of nutrients. It also helps lower the risk of developing cancer of the colon.

Extra bonuses for IBS sufferers are that exercise helps rid your body of excess fluids and tones your abdomen. Toned muscles act like a lycra leotard to hold the stomach in and reduce the effects of bloating and swelling. And because exercise boosts levels of endorphins, body hormones that increase the sense of wellbeing, it is also one of the best ways of easing stress.

## Take action

❑ You don't need to join a gym (unless you want to) and it doesn't matter what kind of exercise you do – walk, jog, swim, cycle, dance, roller blade, play a leisurely game of tennis, the choice is yours. Just make sure it's something you enjoy. The key is to do some kind of activity that makes you feel warm and slightly out of breath for 30 minutes most days of the week.

❑ You should also include some strength exercises using weights, or your own body weight and stretching (for example yoga or Pilates).

❑ If your symptoms are triggered by stress, it may be best to avoid stressful or competitive sports and activities because these can exacerbate symptoms.

# Managing IBS at home

Managing your condition at home is probably easier than anywhere else. You are in your own environment, you can decide what you eat and drink and you know where the toilet is! The main problem may be other people. Research has found that IBS sufferers often feel those close to them don't care for them. It pays to find out as much as you can about your condition, and let your family or living companions know how it affects you and how they can support you in the most helpful way when you experience a flare-up.

## Managing your everyday life

**Slow down** Even if you thrive on stress and excitement, it's no good trying to live at top speed the whole time. Make some time to do things that demand a slower pace. For example, take up an activity like drawing or painting, go for a slow swim or walk rather than a run, or make yoga one of your exercise sessions. Learn to meditate, or make time to stand and stare.

**Change the way you think** People who habitually get anxious and stressed often automatically think negatively about things.

Try to identify negative thoughts and stop them in their tracks. When something gets you down, ask yourself, does it really matter? When facing something stressful, put it into perspective – think about how you will feel about it this time next year or in five years' time.

**Stop catastrophizing** That is, stop thinking that everything is the worst thing that could ever happen. The truth is we all have problems from time to time and few are really catastrophic. Try to regard bad things that happen as opportunities to learn and then move on.

**Learn to laugh** Being able to see the funny side of things helps you to relax.

**Say 'No' to negative thoughts** Many of us tend to focus on what we imagine to be our bad qualities all the time and pay no attention to our good characteristics. Start being kinder to yourself. Congratulate yourself for a job well done. If you do make a mistake, as everyone does from time to time, don't castigate yourself. Think about the things you did right and work out how you might do things differently next time.

# IBS at work

Work can be one of the most difficult environments in which to manage IBS and can in itself be a considerable source of stress. Research shows that the most stressful jobs are those in which you have little control over your work, for example middle management or production line.

Some IBS sufferers feel that they have to give up their jobs because they find it all just too difficult. This is extremely unfortunate because having a job is a great source of self-esteem and self-worth as well as poviding much-needed funds for living and enjoying yourself. With a few adjustments, giving up your job isn't always necessary, except in the most severe cases of IBS.

❑ The options for work are expanding and many more non-routine jobs or patterns of working are available. This is great for people with IBS who may find the nine-to-five stressful. You might consider downsizing, working from home, working part-time or taking a less stressful job within the organization for which you work (if you can afford it).

❑ Make sure your boss and/or personnel manager knows about your condition and how it affects you. It may be possible to make arrangements to work from home or ease off on work during flare-ups.

❑ If you have a choice, position your desk or work-station close to the lavatory.

## GETTING SUPPORT

With any chronic illness, it is vital to have the sympathy and support of those around you. Sympathetic as many of your friends and family may be, perhaps no one can really understand as much as someone who suffers in the same way. You may want to consider joining an IBS self-help group or support network, or join in one of the many chat rooms on the Internet. There you will find people who know what you are going through because they experience it themselves. You may also pick up practical tips to help you manage your condition better.

- Plan your journey to work. Use the lavatory before you go and make sure you know the whereabouts of public toilets en route. If you can, try to travel out of the rush hour so that your journey is less stressful.

- Manage your time. This can be one of the most important things you can do to alleviate workplace stress. Tackle high-priority jobs first and at a time of day when you feel most alert (for many people this is first thing in the morning), delay or delegate less urgent or non-essential jobs and learn to say 'No'.

- Make sure you get regular breaks during the working day. Have a walk around every hour or so, make yourself a herbal tea, have a chat with a colleague or take a few minutes to stretch and look about.

- Take time out during your working day to relax. Go for a walk in the park or a green open space during your lunch hour if there is one nearby, or try to fit in some exercise.

- If you find yourself getting stressed at work, drop your shoulders, take a deep sighing breath and spend a few minutes with your eyelids gently closed breathing slowly.

## Travelling with IBS

Travel can be a challenge for IBS sufferers, partly because of the stress of having to be somewhere on time and the inevitable delays and cancellations. There's also the worry about finding a lavatory in an unfamiliar place, especially if urgency and diarrhoea are dominant symptoms. If you're travelling by car, look at a map beforehand to see where service areas are. You might like to contact your motor organization for details of pubs, hotels and facilities.

When travelling by plane or train, always request a seat that is close to the toilet. Once you arrive at your destination, immediately have a good look round or get a plan of the place you are visiting and check out shopping areas, hotels and restaurants. If you are travelling abroad, make sure that you find the expression, 'Is there a toilet?' in your phrase book, and you should also ensure that you have the necessary small change for using the toilet.

Wherever you're travelling it always makes sense to carry a small packet of tissues or wet wipes in case there's no toilet paper available. Finally, if the worst comes to the worst and there aren't any public toilets close by, don't be shy – a explanation that you aren't well is all that will be required.

## Eating on holiday

The chance to sample different cuisines is one of the great joys of travelling, but food can be a big issue. One possible solution is to buy a recipe book for the country you are visiting and go self-catering, so that you have control over what you eat.

IBS often comes on after a bout of traveller's tummy or food poisoning, and certainly it can make existing symptoms worse. To avoid a stomach upset, observe the following precautions, especially if you are travelling outside western Europe, North America and Australia:

❑ Drink only bottled or boiled water (for example in hot drinks like teas)

❑ Avoid ice in drinks

❑ Don't brush your teeth with tap water

❑ If you can't avoid unsterilized water, buy water-sterilizing tablets from adventure shops and pharmacies

- ❏ Avoid salads, buffets and uncooked food and peel fruit before eating
- ❏ Make sure hot meals are really piping hot and haven't been allowed to stand
- ❏ Avoid street foods and steer clear of anything you know upsets you, such as spicy or fatty foods.

If you are unfortunate enough to go down with a bout of traveller's tummy:

- ❏ use packs of rehydration mix, available from pharmacies – pack some in your luggage just in case
- ❏ drink plenty of bottled or sterilized water, soft drinks or fruit juices (if you can tolerate them) to combat dehydration
- ❏ light foods, such as boiled rice, are usually well-tolerated; steer clear of complicated dishes and spicy foods until you are better
- ❏ If you experience severe diarrhoea, fever or chills, or there is blood in your stools, seek medical help.

# 3 The orthodox medical approach

You may be able to keep your irritable bowel under control yourself by following the self-help tips outlined in the last chapter. However, there are likely to be times when it is helpful to have active medical treatment. Although he or she will not be able to cure your IBS, your doctor will be able to suggest medications that can help bring your symptoms under control. He or she may also offer you practical tips on the best way to manage your condition, and give reassurance that your symptoms are not caused by anything serious or life threatening.

There is a tremendous range of medications available for IBS, both over-the-counter and on prescription. The ones your doctor recommends will depend on the precise nature of your symptoms and whether diarrhoea or constipation is the more troublesome condition.

This huge choice means it is likely that, with a little trial and error, you and your doctor will be able to find a treatment regimen that helps ease your symptoms and allows you to lead a fuller life. You may not need medication all the time, but the knowledge that it is there if you need it can do much to foster a sense of security.

## When to see the doctor

If your symptoms are mild and do not bother you unduly, it may not be necessary to consult your doctor. However, if the symptoms are persistent and are seriously disrupting your life, if they are especially severe or if you develop symptoms for the first time when you are over the age of 45, it is worth making an appointment. This is especially important if you notice blood in your motions. Many people find that they worry less about their condition after they have seen a doctor, which can only help improve symptoms in itself.

## Getting a diagnosis

Medical consultations tend to follow a set pattern: first the doctor will ask for a detailed medical history which includes symptoms of the problem you are seeking help for, then he or she will perform a physical examination and, where necessary, perform or recommend one or more tests to either confirm or refute diagnosis.

You will get the most out of your consultation if you go prepared with any information your doctor is likely to require. The doctor may do some tests to rule out serious causes, but in the first instance is likely to rely on the information you provide to make a diagnosis.

# Your medical history

Typically, this will include questions about the following areas:

☐ diseases and operations you have had in the past

☐ any diseases that run in your family

☐ your general health

☐ your eating and drinking habits

☐ whether you smoke

☐ the kind of work you do

☐ how much physical activity you get

☐ your irritable bowel syndrome

This information will help your doctor to determine the most likely cause of your symptoms so that he or she can prescribe you the most appropriate medication, where necessary, and offer you the most appropriate advice on management.

Specifically, the doctor is likely to ask you a set of questions based on an internationally agreed system for diagnosing IBS, which is known as the Rome Criteria. The questions are designed to identify IBS and distinguish it from other bowel disorders. They include:

1 In the past three months, have you experienced continuous or recurrent abdominal pain or discomfort which is:

☐ relieved by opening your bowels?

☐ linked with a change in frequency of opening your bowels?

☐ linked with a change in consistency of your bowel movements?

2 Have you experienced two or more of the following on at least a quarter of occasions:

☐ changed frequency of bowel movements?

- changed consistency of bowel motions, for example more lumpy and hard or more loose and watery?
- alterations in bowel movements, for example straining, a desperate need to open your bowels or feeling of incomplete emptying?
- bloating or a feeling of fullness?

The more times you answered 'Yes', the more likely it is that you have irritable bowel syndrome.

# Tests that may be done

Because IBS is a functional disease, that is one that doesn't cause any detectable physical changes, there is no specific test the doctor can use to make a definitive diagnosis. Instead, he or she will have to rely on your description of the pattern of symptoms and may also do some tests that are designed to rule out other diseases with similar symptoms. The exact tests done will depend on how long you have had IBS, your age and the symptoms you are experiencing.

## Abdominal palpation

The doctor will probably ask you to lie down so that he or she can palpate your abdomen (feel it with his or her hands) to check for tenderness or swellings. In IBS there will usually be nothing to feel apart possibly from slight tenderness if your abdomen is distended.

## Rectal examination

You may then be asked to lie on your side so that your doctor can carry out a rectal examination. This involves inserting a lubricated, gloved finger into your rectum to check for any swellings or abnormalities which could indicate a more serious condition. Although slightly undignified, this is not at all painful. In IBS the rectum is completely normal.

## Blood test

The doctor will also take a blood sample to check for anaemia and analyse your blood chemistry for any signs of infection.

# Referral to a specialist

In some cases, for example if you are over 45 and have developed symptoms for the first time, the doctor may refer you to a specialist gastroenterologist (a doctor trained and experienced in the diagnosis and treatment of gastrointestinal diseases and problems) for further tests. You will receive an appointment to attend a gastrointestinal clinic. The tests you have will depend on your symptoms. For instance, if diarrhoea is a major symptom, the specialist may recommend stool sampling for infections and sometimes tests for malabsorption. If you are over 50, the doctor will usually recommend sigmoidoscopy or colonoscopy. Tests may include the ones already described, plus one or more of those detailed below.

If you fit the criteria for IBS and the investigations above don't suggest signs of other disease, the doctor is likely to give you a diagnosis of IBS.

## Stool sampling

A sample of your stool is examined for evidence of viral, bacterial or parasitic infection, which can lead to diarrhoea and vomiting. It will also be examined for evidence of occult (hidden) blood, which may be an early sign of bowel cancer.

## Sigmoidoscopy

This involves using an instrument called a sigmoidoscope, a soft, flexible viewing tube with a light at its tip to examine the lining of the rectum and lower colon for bleeding, inflammation or unusual swellings.

You'll be asked to lie on your left side. The doctor will then gently insert the sigmoidoscope through your anus and into your colon. The sigmoidoscope blows air into the colon to keep the walls of the bowel apart so the doctor can view them

---

## BEFORE YOU VISIT THE DOCTOR

Make a note of the following to help your doctor make a diagnosis:

1 When your symptoms first developed
2 Any factors associated with the onset of symptoms, such as eating particular foods, stress, travel, time of day and so on
3 The pattern of your symptoms: when they tend to come on, how long they last, whether they come and go or are continuous
4 Anything that eases symptoms, such as having a bowel movement
5 What treatments or self-help measures you have already tried, including drugs, medicines and any complementary treatments
6 Whether the pattern of your symptoms has changed recently
7 Any particular questions or concerns you may have.

---

more easily. Although this is uncomfortable rather than painful, it can trigger IBS-like symptoms of pressure, wind, bloating or cramping. The whole procedure takes between about five and twenty minutes. If the doctor finds any abnormalities, he or she may remove a small sample of tissue to be sent for analysis.

You will be asked to abstain from solid food for 12–24 hours before the procedure, and may be given one or more enemas to ensure the colon and rectum are completely empty.

## Colonoscopy

This is an investigation that is similar to sigmoidoscopy. A colonoscope, a longer flexible tube around 1 m (3¼ ft) in length, which is used by the doctor to examine the lining of the whole of the bowel for abnormalities. A biopsy (tissue sample) may be taken, if necessary, to check out any abnormalities.

You will be given a laxative the day before the examination and asked to abstain from eating and drinking for six hours before the procedure takes place. The procedure is carried out under local anaesthetic. Afterwards, you'll be allowed to rest or doze until the effects of the anaesthetic have worn off sufficiently to enable you to go home. You won't be allowed to drive, so you should make arrangements for someone to accompany you home.

## Lower gastrointestinal x-ray (barium enema)

This is an extremely common test used to diagnose lower gastrointestinal problems, such as abnormal growths, ulcers, polyps and other swellings. A thick liquid, containing the compound barium sulphate, is given by means of an enema to coat the lining of the colon and rectum. The barium shows up on x-ray, enabling the examiner to see the shape and size of your bowel and any abnormalities.

A barium enema can be somewhat uncomfortable and cause IBS-like feelings of swelling and pressure. You may feel the urge to open your bowels, although it is not possible for this to actually happen as the enema used to inject the barium has a balloon on the end that prevents the ejection of liquid. You'll be allowed to empty your bowels after the procedure is completed. The procedure usually takes between one or two hours in total.

The barium will be expelled over the next few bowel motions. It can cause constipation and make your faeces white or grey for a few days afterwards.

To prepare for the procedure, you will probably be asked to drink only clear liquids the night before and take a laxative to clear out your bowel.

## Lactose tolerance test

Lactase is an enzyme produced by the small intestine that breaks down lactose or milk sugar. If you lack this enzyme, either because you were born with a lactase deficiency or following an episode of gastroenteritis, your body will be unable to digest milk and milk products such as cheese and yogurt.

Lactase deficiency can cause symptoms of bloating, diarrhoea, abdominal pain and wind similar to IBS. The doctor may want to perform a lactose tolerance test to see how well your body breaks down lactose in the intestines.

You will be asked to abstain from eating and drinking for eight to twelve hours and a blood sample will be taken from your fingertip to measure the amount of sugar in your blood. You will then be given a solution containing milk sugar and lemon to drink.

If your body is breaking down lactose as it should, the level of blood sugar will rise within an hour. If this does not

## IMPORTANT REASONS TO SEE THE DOCTOR

Although it is rare for intestinal symptoms to indicate anything serious, in some instances some of the symptoms associated with IBS may be signs of other potentially more serious illness that needs treatment. You should consult your doctor without delay if:

○ you notice blood in your stools
○ your stools are black
○ you develop a raised temperature and experience abdominal pain
○ you are losing weight for no apparent reason and you are not on a diet
○ you experience severe and prolonged abdominal pain that is sufficient to wake you from a deep sleep or cause vomiting
○ you notice blood or black clots in your vomit
○ you have a family history of bowel cancer
○ you develop symptoms of IBS for the first time after the age of 45

happen, it may mean that lactose is not being processed properly. This may be due to a lack of the enzyme lactase which breaks down lactose.

## Medications for IBS

Once the doctor has all the information needed, he or she may write you a prescription. Your doctor will also offer you practical suggestions on your lifestyle to help you manage your condition more effectively and reduce the severity of your symptoms and the number of acute attacks.

There are several distinct forms of treatment that may play a part in your overall treatment plan. These can include laxatives, fibre supplements, antispasmodic drugs, antacids and preparations for the treatment of wind, anti-diarrhoeal medications, smooth muscle relaxants and in some cases anti-depressants.

None of the medications will actually make your irritable bowel syndrome go away for good, but they can help reduce pain and discomfort and control symptoms such as diarrhoea and constipation.

## Tailoring treatment to you

Just as the symptoms of IBS can vary in severity from person to person and from day to day, so there is a spectrum of treatments available. The doctor will try as far as possible to tailor treatment to you as an individual.

There is no one guaranteed treatment for IBS and it can often take quite a large amount of trial and error to find the treatment or treatments that work best for you. If you find that a treatment you are prescribed is not effective, do not be afraid to go back to the doctor and request further help. It will often be possible to prescribe a different treatment that works better for you.

Always inform your doctor if you experience any problems or side-effects after taking medications you have been prescribed or have purchased yourself over the counter. Many sufferers find a combination of several different treatments aimed at different symptoms works better than one single treatment. Others prefer to try to manage without medication most of the time but to have medications that they know work for them on hand in case symptoms become overwhelming or unmanageable.

# Psychotherapy

Because IBS can be so closely related to stress, psychotherapy can often be a particularly successful treatment. One type of psychotherapy that is widely used and often as helpful as drugs and medications is cognitive behavioural therapy. This aims to help you identify and correct patterns of faulty thinking, both in your life generally and in relation to your irritable bowel in particular.

For example, you might think, 'I'll never be able to go anywhere or do anything because of my irritable bowel.' This thought can lead to stress, anxiety and depression, and intensify symptoms. Cognitive behavioural therapy teaches you to pinpoint such negative thoughts and replace them with more realistic, positive ones. For example, you might be encouraged to replace the initial thought with, 'Okay so my irritable bowel does make it more difficult to plan things, but with some forethought it doesn't have to incapacitate me.'

During a course of cognitive behavioural therapy, you learn exercises and strategies to help you feel more in control of your life and symptoms, and to challenge beliefs which may be stopping you from living life as fully as you can.

## Group therapy

Some specialists run group therapy sessions for people with IBS. This usually involves a series of meetings, looking at how the gut works and the role various factors such as diet and stress may play in IBS. They will also encourage people to take control of their condition by doing various psychological exercises and relaxation.

# TREATMENTS FOR DIARRHOEA

These either act on the bowel wall to slow down its contractions or alter the consistency of the stool.

| Drugs | How they act | Watchpoint |
|---|---|---|
| **Drugs that slow bowel contractions** | | |
| **e.g. Loperamide** | These slow the peristaltic wave, increase bowel transit and reduce intestinal hurry and diarrhoea. They are used to help diarrhoea, urgency and abdominal pain. They also help increase the tone of the sphincter, the ring of muscle that keeps the rectum closed until you want to open your bowels. Some products can be bought over the counter: they are often advertised for the relief of 'holiday tummy'. | ○ Can cause rash, stomach cramps, bloating and constipation.<br>○ Don't use if you are breastfeeding or pregnant, or if you suffer from kidney failure, dysentery or blocked intestine.<br>○ These drugs belong to the opiate family, and although they do not cross the blood-brain barrier, they can, in some cases, lead to dependency. |
| **Drugs that alter stool consistency** | | |
| **e.g. Ispaghula husk** | These are all bulking agents. They may come in the form of effervescent granules, powder or tablets. They work by absorbing excess fluid from the stool as it passes through the gut. This produces a larger stool and can prevent spasms. | ○ Bulking agents don't work for everyone and in some cases actually aggravate diarrhoea.<br>○ Do not use if you have kidney, circulatory or heart problems, blocked intestines or inelastic colon.<br>○ Other medications that can help include kaolin, charcoal, chalk and pectin. They work by combining with excess fluid in the stool. |

# TREATMENTS FOR CONSTIPATION

**There are a number of different types of laxatives. They include bulking agents, osmotic laxatives, stimulant laxatives and stool softeners.**

| Drugs | How they act | Watchpoint |
|---|---|---|
| **Bulking agents** | | |
| e.g. Ispaghula husk | As already described, these drugs work by absorbing water from the gut, making the stools bulkier, softer and easier to pass. Because they are gentle, they are the safest type of laxative. It is worth bearing in mind that these products usually take several days to work. | ○ Although safe and gentle generally, the sensitive guts of people with IBS do not always tolerate these drugs and symptoms such as pain, bloating, wind and diarrhoea may worsen. |
| **Osmotic laxatives** | | |
| e.g. Lactulose, magnesium hydroxide | These are solutions of mineral salts or sugars (usually sodium, magnesium or potassium), which work by drawing water into the gut to soften and loosen the stools. The water triggers peristalsis, which speeds up gut transit time. They include many over-the-counter remedies. | ○ Take with plenty of water to avoid dehydration. <br> ○ Can trigger wind, stomach cramps and abdominal pain. <br> ○ May interact with antacids and the antibiotic niomycin. <br> ○ Lactulose-based osmotics are often poorly tolerated by people with IBS. They can cause nausea, wind, cramps, flatulence and bloating. Lactulose shouldn't be used by people with the inherited enzyme disorder galacto-saemia, or people with blocked intestine. <br> ○ Osmotics containing magnesium should not be used by people with kidney problems. <br> ○ Osmotics containing sodium should not be used by people with high blood pressure, or heart, liver or kidney problems. |

# TREATMENTS FOR CONSTIPATION

There are a number of different types of laxatives. They include bulking agents, osmotic laxatives, stimulant laxatives and stool softeners.

| Drugs | How they act | Watchpoint |
|---|---|---|
| **Stimulant laxatives** | | |
| **e.g. Senna pods, bisacodyl, sterculia** | These work by irritating the walls of the gut, stimulating it to contract powerfully and propel the stool through the intestine. They usually take between six and twelve hours to work. | ○ Because they are irritating, these drugs can cause stomach cramps and abdominal pain in the sensitive guts of people with IBS.<br>○ Some types should not be taken within an hour of taking antacids.<br>○ Some types should not be taken at bedtime.<br>○ Prolonged use should be avoided as repeated use can eventually damage the bowel.<br>○ Not to be used with intestinal blockage, impacted faeces or inelastic colon. |
| **Stool softeners** | | |
| **e.g. Docusate sodium** | As the name suggests, these drugs act to soften the stools, allowing the bowel to propel the stools on faster and make them easier to pass. They work by breaking up surface tension of the stool in a similar way to detergent. | ○ Stool softeners take a day or so to act.<br>○ Some kinds are best avoided if you are pregnant or breastfeeding, and should not be used if there is intestinal obstruction. |

# TREATMENTS FOR PAIN, WIND AND BLOATING

| Drugs | How they act | Watchpoint |
|---|---|---|
| **Anti-spasmodic drugs** | | |
| **e.g. Mebeverin, alverine citrate, hyoscine butylbromide** | Widely prescribed for the relief of IBS, anti-spasmodics are designed to prevent spasms of the bowel walls that cause abdominal pain. They work by decreasing the abnormal sensitivity of receptors in the smooth muscle of the gut and are especially useful for the relief of abdominal pain. Although studies have shown that these drugs can reduce abdominal pain and urgency, it's not certain how effective they are in the long term. | ○ Some anti-spasmodics can cause dry mouth, blurred vision, confusion and problems passing urine.<br>○ Mebeverin should not be used by people with intestinal block or porphyria.<br>○ Alverine citrate should not be used in pregnancy.<br>○ Hyoscine butyl-bromide should not be used if you have glaucoma, intestinal obstruction or inflammation, or an enlarged prostate. |
| **Peppermint oil products** | | |
| **e.g. Peppermint oil** | Peppermint oil contains menthol, which helps relax the smooth muscle of the gut. Some people find the oil and other peppermint-based medications help ease pain, wind and bloating. | ○ Some products may very occasionally cause heartburn, allergy, rash, headache, irregular heartbeat or tremors.<br>○ Caution is needed with antacids. |

# OTHER TREATMENTS

| Drugs | How they act | Watchpoint |
|---|---|---|
| **Anti-depressants** | | |
| **e.g. Tricyclic anti-depressants (e.g. amitriptyline, imipramine, and despramine) or selective serotonin reuptake inhibitors (e.g. fluoxetine, sertraline, and paroxetine)** | Your doctor may treat you with anti-depressants known as tricyclics, or with one of the newer selective serotonin reuptake inhibitors (SSRIs) which boost levels of serotonin, the happiness hormone, in the brain. This hormone is the subject of a great deal of interest for the part it may play in IBS. Research has found that anti-depressants can alleviate symptoms independent of their primary (anti-depressive) effects. It is not known exactly why this is the case, although it is almost certainly related to the brain-gut connection. It could be that they work on the bowel wall to decrease contractions and spasm. Alternatively, they may decrease pain or the perception of pain from intestinal spasm. | ○ It can take four to six weeks before an improvement in symptoms is experienced.<br>○ Tricyclic anti-depressants can cause dry mouth, blurred vision and difficulty passing urine. They can also cause constipation.<br>○ Other side-effects may include nausea, vomiting, headache, anxiety, insomnia, dizziness, drowsiness, rash and, more rarely, mania (hyperactive behaviour).<br>○ You should only take them on the advice of a doctor if you are pregnant, have epilepsy, liver or kidney problems, heart disease or diabetes. You shouldn't take them if you are breastfeeding or suffering unstable epilepsy.<br>○ Some SSRIs can interact with other drugs, including some other anti-depressants. |

# 4 Help from complementary therapies

Complementary therapies are growing in popularity, especially among people with chronic conditions like IBS which aren't easily treated by orthodox methods. One study of 225 IBS patients at London's Royal London School of Medicine found that half of all IBS patients had consulted a complementary therapist for help with their condition.

In part these findings may reflect the difficulty and frustration many people with IBS feel in their dealings with conventional doctors.

Using complementary therapies can help you to feel more in control of your condition, especially where there is no clear-cut treatment or cure. Many people with IBS find a combination of complementary therapies and conventional treatment is the most effective way to control symptoms.

However, it is important not to expect complementary therapy to be a miracle cure. As we've seen time and again so far in this book, there is no single solution to IBS, so it's a question of finding what methods best suit you.

## How complementary therapies can help

Unlike orthodox medicine, which tends to focus mainly on symptoms, complementary therapies address health problems as part of a larger picture that includes diet, lifestyle and beliefs as well as symptoms: that is, they are holistic. Before treating you, a complementary therapist will want to know a lot about you and your lifestyle. This is particularly relevant with regard to IBS because, as we've seen, patterns of symptoms are often closely related to other aspects of lifestyle.

Another important way in which complementary therapies can be useful is that many of them work by helping to induce relaxation. Again, as already outlined, this can be an extremely valuable tool in helping to control symptoms.

There is a whole range of complementary therapies that people have found useful in managing irritable bowel, some of which are described below. Hypnotherapy, in particular, has been studied in a number of clinical trials and as a result is gaining the respect of a growing number of orthodox doctors as a means of helping to relieve stress and control the symptoms of IBS.

Do bear in mind that although the therapies detailed have been found to be helpful by some people, most of them haven't undergone the same kind of controlled trials that conventional medical treatments have and they aren't the only therapies that may be useful. No single treatment is right for everyone, so when seeking treatment, it is very largely a question of trial and error and experimenting to find what works best for you.

## Complementary medicine – is it safe, does it work?

Because most complementary medical treatments have not been assessed by carrying out the same rigorous scientifically controlled trials that conventional treatments have to undergo, it can be difficult to evaluate how safe or effective they are. Supporters of complementary treatments tend to point to the fact that they have stood the test of time. However, this in itself is not proof of safety or efficacy. Unfortunately, because many trials into orthodox treatments are funded by pharmaceutical companies, research into complementary therapies tends to be underfunded. Also, trials can be difficult to conduct because the therapies themselves are often individualized so that different patients with the same condition receive different treatments.

For these reasons, some orthodox doctors are cautious about recommending complementary therapies. The good news is that an increasing amount of research is now being done and evidence is accumulating that a number of complementary treatments can be useful in helping to manage certain conditions, among them IBS.

## Active therapies

Hypnotherapy, yoga and meditation are all therapies that involve you in some sort of active participation – for example, controlling your breathing, thoughts or movement, or visualizing your gut becoming less active. Although the therapies differ in their specific approach, what they have in common is a belief that what happens in the mind affects the body. Orthodox practitioners have begun to take this guiding principle seriously in recent years, with the discovery of brain chemicals and receptors in the gut. In fact, the emerging discipline of neuro-gastroenterology is concerned specifically with the links between the brain and the gastrointestinal tract.

## Hypnotherapy

Hypnotherapy is practised all over the world as a method of treating both physical and emotional problems and those which, like irritable bowel, have aspects of the two. In the past decade or so, a number of influential research studies have been conducted into the effects of hypnotherapy on the symptoms of IBS.

Hypnotherapy acts to deeply relax your body and focus your mind. In a hypnotic state or trance, your body is in a state of complete relaxation, similar to that achieved under meditation and akin to the moment before you fall asleep. In this state, a number of bodily functions controlled by the autonomic nervous system – the part of your nervous system that controls functions that are outside your conscious control such as your breathing, heart rate, metabolism and the activity of the gut – slow down just as they do when you are asleep. At the same time, your mind is highly receptive and this can be used to help change the way you think or feel.

Of all the complementary therapies, hypnotherapy is the one that has received the most support from the orthodox medical profession as a treatment for IBS. In fact, studies suggest that hypnotherapy improves symptoms in some eight out of ten sufferers with classic IBS symptoms – abdominal pain, bloating, frequency and constipation or diarrhoea – and without additional complicating factors such as depression.

One of the first and most significant studies, conducted in Manchester in the 1980s, showed that hypnotherapy effected a dramatic reduction in IBS symptoms in people who had failed to respond to orthodox medical treatment. Since then, a number of other studies conducted in the UK and the US have mirrored these results. The precise way in which hypnotherapy works to reduce IBS symptoms as yet remains a mystery, although several studies have shown that it can slow bowel transit time, reduce the secretion of stomach acids and calm gut motility.

**What to expect** There are a number of different methods used to induce the hypnotic state but in essence they all involve helping you to relax. One widely used method involves the hypnotherapist asking you to concentrate on a real or imagined object while breathing slowly in and out. Once you are fully relaxed, the therapist may encourage you to visualize a beautiful scene to help you relax more deeply and to encourage your mind to focus. While you are in the hypnotic state, the therapist may use suggestion or guided imagery to help you become calm and begin to deal with problems that are bothering you.

## Gut-directed hypnotherapy
In gut-directed hypnotherapy, the emphasis is specifically on the symptoms of IBS and on helping you control the

movements of your gut. You will be given information on how the gut functions and the relationship between the mind and the gut. While you are in a hypnotic state, the therapist may ask you to imagine the muscles in your gut relaxing or encourage you to imagine a river flowing smoothly along to help you address your symptoms. At the end of the session, the therapist will help you to work your way back to consciousness. You will usually be encouraged to learn self-hypnosis using a tape at home. Researchers have claimed results in as few as seven sessions, although thirteen including the initial consultation is the norm.

## Yoga

Yoga – the word means 'union' in Sanskrit – is a system that aims to unite the body and the mind and to restore balance to both. There are many different forms of yoga, but the one that is most widely practised in the West – and the type that forms the basis of most yoga classes – is hatha yoga. The main purpose of hatha yoga is to achieve unity by means of practising physical postures (asanas), breathing (pranayama) and meditation (dhyana).

According to ancient yogic principles, breathing correctly (pranayama) is the way to control all mental and bodily functions. Modern Western research has also confirmed the importance of breathing. Most of us tend to breathe too shallowly in our upper chest and do not make use of the full capacity of our lungs. Yogic breathing encourages the full use of the whole lungs by bringing a greater awareness of how you breathe through a series of exercises designed to help you control your breath.

Many of the asanas or postures in yoga are designed to massage and relax the internal organs in a way that conventional exercise techniques do not.

Yoga is particularly helpful in alleviating stress-related conditions, and although there haven't been any scientific trials specifically on the use of yoga for IBS, several studies have found that stress commonly triggers symptoms in people who are susceptible.

**What to expect**  Yoga is often taught in classes lasting for an hour or so. If you've never done a class before, go for a beginner's class or drop-in session which will be geared to people of different levels. The postures are done in bare feet and you should wear loose, comfortable clothes that allow you to move freely. A yoga mat will usually be supplied, but you may like to buy your own after a few sessions.

Before the class, the teacher will usually ask if anyone has any particular health problems, but if he or she doesn't ask, you should mention it. A typical session usually starts with five or ten minutes of relaxation and breathing awareness while lying down, followed by a series of asanas or postures, designed to stretch and relax your muscles. The teacher will demonstrate these and talk you through them.

It takes time to become supple enough to do all the postures and you will probably find that some come more easily than others. Make sure that you work to your own level and concentrate on what you are doing – don't compare yourself with the person next to you or others in the class. Each session usually ends with another brief relaxation session which may include some meditation or chanting.

## Meditation and visualization

Meditation is used throughout the world in many different cultures and religions to achieve a state of calm consciousness. It is part of Buddhism, Hinduism and Christianity. Like hypnosis, it involves focusing the mind to attain a state of alert relaxation. A relaxed mind produces significant physical benefits. It has been found that regular meditation can slow the heart rate, lower blood pressure, regulate breathing and balance the metabolism. It also helps reduce levels of the stress hormone, adrenaline, which is involved in the flight or fight reaction and is particularly relevant in irritable bowel.

**What to expect** There is no one way to meditate, so you should ask the group leader what the technique involves or go to a session to find out for yourself. You can meditate by sitting or kneeling quietly and focusing on your breath or on an object such as a flower, a pebble or a candle. Some techniques encourage you to focus on a mantra, a word or sound such as the Sanskrit word 'om' or 'peace'. Other techniques use chanting or singing.

Visualization, in which you are encouraged to focus on a real or imagined image or scene, is one of the most commonly used techniques. It is common for the conscious mind to resist attempts to turn it off and you are likely to find that intrusive thoughts interfere with your attempts to meditate. You will be encouraged to observe them and let them go. Meditation works best when practised regularly.

## Relaxation and biofeedback training

Learning to relax, as described in Chapter 2, pages 43–45 is one of the most useful ways in which you can help yourself manage

IBS. Biofeedback training uses electronic instruments to help you monitor how relaxed you are and control your physical reactions. As with hypnotherapy, the technique may be used both to achieve general relaxation or to specifically address bowel symptoms.

A number of studies have been conducted into biofeedback, and it is beginning to emerge as one of the most promising complementary treatments for IBS. In one study conducted at London's Royal Free Hospital, 40 IBS patients used a computer-aided biofeedback game and were asked to keep a diary of symptoms. Half the patients experienced a reduction in symptoms. Biofeedback can also be used to help sufferers in whom constipation is a problem by helping them relax their pelvic floor muscles during bowel movements. Other techniques involve the use of an electronic stethoscope to feedback bowel sounds. The sufferer uses relaxation techniques to try and control these sounds and hence their bowel activity.

**What to expect** Biofeedback is increasingly being used in physiotherapy departments and departments of psychiatry and gastroenterology in hospitals. In a biofeedback session, relaxation techniques similar to those already described in Chapter 2, pages 44–45, are taught. Sensors are attached to your body and connected to a machine or computer that allows you to monitor bodily responses such as heart rate, temperature, muscle tension or bowel sounds. Whatever method is used, the aim is to enable you to learn how to control your physical reactions and so reduce symptoms. Once you have learned how to relax, you can dispense with the machine and induce relaxation at will.

# Natural therapies

Natural therapies, such as homoeopathy, herbalism and naturopathy, are complete systems of therapy which aim to enlist the body's own self-healing mechanisms to cure illness and enhance health and wellbeing.

## Homoeopathy

Homoeopathy was developed in the 19th century by German physician Samuel Hahnemann and is now one of the most popular complementary therapies. The remedies are based on the principle that like treats like. This means that a substance that causes symptoms of disease in a healthy person will cure the same or similar symptoms in someone who is unwell. This is the opposite of orthodox medicine where illnesses are treated with their antidote.

So for example, when treating diarrhoea, an orthodox doctor would prescribe a medication that induces constipation, whereas a homoeopathic practitioner would prescribe a minute dose of a substance that would provoke diarrhoea if used in a larger dose. The idea behind this is to stimulate the body's own self-healing mechanism.

Homoeopathic remedies are prepared by diluting substances from animal, vegetable and mineral sources in a 'mother tincture' of alcohol and water until there is no detectable active ingredient left. Between dilutions, the mixture is succussed or shaken. This process is believed to transfer some of the vital energy or 'vibrational pattern' of the natural ingredient into the tincture. It is thought that it is this, rather than any chemical ingredient, that stimulates the body's healing mechanism.

## HOMOEOPATHIC REMEDIES FOR IBS

| Remedies | Symptoms |
| --- | --- |
| Belladonna, colocynth, mag. | Abdominal pain and cramps |
| Phos, bryonia alba | Nausea and pain |
| Colchichum Argentum nit | Flatulence and alternating diarrhoea and constipation with mucus in the stools |

Note: Because IBS is a complex condition, it is best not to try to treat yourself but to consult a qualified homoeopathic practitioner.

Homoeopathic remedies are graded into potencies according to how much they have been diluted. A 1c dilution contains one drop of active ingredient added to 99 drops of alcohol and water mix which has been succussed. To get a remedy of the 6c potency (the most commonly available in health food stores and pharmacies) this is done six times. The drops are added to tiny lactose (milk sugar) pills, granules or powder.

**What to expect** An initial consultation is likely to last an hour or an hour and a half. Homoeopathic remedies are prescribed for the whole person, so rather than simply noting your symptoms, the homoeopath will seek details about you as a person, your personality, your likes and dislikes and your responses to your environment. For example, he or she might ask whether your symptoms are better for heat or cold, what kind of food your prefer – hot, cold, sweet, sour or savoury – previous illnesses, and any family medical problems. Armed with this information, the homoeopath will prescribe the remedy that most closely matches the picture built up of you and your symptoms. No two people with IBS will be treated alike.

Remedies are prescribed one at a time, so you may be prescribed one remedy to be taken for three or four days, followed by another. Remedies should be taken in a clean mouth – no tea, coffee, alcohol or toothpaste – and allowed to dissolve under the tongue. Symptoms tend to disappear in the reverse order in which they appeared.

## Herbalism

Herbs have been used for healing all over the world since ancient times. Indeed many modern drugs derive from the numerous different compounds that are found in herbs. Herbalism is part of the Western medical tradition and is also known to be part of the heritage of Africa, India, China and the Americas as well.

When herbs are used in their whole form as bark, leaves, seeds, roots and flowers, as they are in herbalism, they contain a host of different chemicals. Many of these chemicals act to balance the effects of others and so reduce the danger of unwelcome side-effects.

Both Western herbalism and Chinese herbal treatments have been subjected to scientific trials and are looking extremely promising in the treatment of IBS.

In one study, a modified preparation of a herbal tincture known as Iberogast – a blend of clown's mustard, camomile, angelica, caraway, milk thistle, melissa, celandine, licorice and peppermint – was tested on 157 IBS sufferers. Those taking the modified preparation experienced a significant improvement in abdominal pain and other symptoms.

## Western herbalism

Western herbalism combines the traditional knowledge of herbs with modern scientific developments. Medical herbalists

## HERBS FOR IBS

| Symptoms | Useful herbs |
| --- | --- |
| **Irritated digestive tract** | Comfrey, hops, marshmallow, oats, slippery elm |
| **Wind and flatulence** | Angelica, aniseed, caraway, cayenne, German camomile, dill, fennel, ginger, thyme, peppermint |
| **Diarrhoea** | Meadowsweet, arrowroot |
| **Constipation** | Barbery, psyllium, dandelion, linseeds, liquorice, yellow dock |
| **Cramp or colic** | German camomile, valerian, lemon balm, ginger, wild yam |

trained in the West are thoroughly versed in anatomy and physiology as well as having a knowledge of the various herbs and how they can be used.

**What to expect** At a first consultation, the herbalist will take a full medical history and ask you questions about your lifestyle, such as your reaction to stress, sleeping and eating patterns, previous illnesses and any medicines you are taking.

Sometimes, though not always, this is followed by a physical examination which may include palpating your abdomen for inflammation and bowel tone. After this, he or she will prescribe a herb or sometimes a combination of herbs and will also give you advice on diet, exercise and relaxation. As well as herbs aimed at specific IBS symptoms, the herbalist may prescribe herbs designed to tackle other associated problems, for example hypericum (St John's Wort) for any underlying depression, valerian or skullcap to calm the nerves and reduce anxiety, and agnus vitex castus or evening primrose oil for IBS associated with PMS.

**Using herbal remedies** Herbs may be prescribed in various forms. These include:

- ❑ Tinctures made by soaking herbs in alcohol to extract and preserve their ingredients.
- ❑ Infusions or herbal teas made by steeping dried herbs in boiling water for 10–15 minutes.
- ❑ Decoctions made by boiling the tougher parts of herbs, such as roots, bark, nuts and seeds, in water before straining and drinking.
- ❑ Tablets and capsules in which the herbs are crushed and taken in the same way as conventional drugs.
- ❑ Creams and ointments used externally.
- ❑ Hot or cold compresses made by soaking a clean piece of cotton in a herbal infusion.
- ❑ Poultices, which are made by crushing fresh herbs or dried herbs moistened into a paste with hot water, applied to the body.
- ❑ Suppositories ready-made to insert, or douches made from infusions or decoctions.
- ❑ Herbal baths which are made by tying a handful of herbs in a muslin bag and hanging it in the bath, or by using aromatherapy oils.

## Aromatherapy

The use of essential oils in massage, inhalations or in the bath can be helpful for IBS sufferers, especially for relaxation purposes. Useful oils include bergamot and grapefruit. It is important that all essential oils are diluted in a carrier oil before massaging, since they are too strong to be applied directly to the skin.

## Massage

Massage uses the power of touch to help you relax and alleviate mental and physical tension that you may feel. It forms part of many complementary therapies, including aromatherapy and naturopathy, and is also part of Ayurvedic medicine and traditional Chinese medicine.

There are many different types of massage but what they all have in common is that they aim to promote relaxation and help regulate breathing, slow the heart rate, lower blood pressure and improve circulation. This makes it particularly useful for stress and stress-linked problems such as IBS.

Techniques include stroking, kneading, pressing with the fingers or knuckles and pummelling. The therapist may use essential oils or a base oil such as almond to help his or her hands glide more smoothly over your body.

## Naturopathy

Naturopathy is a healthcare system that makes use of only natural resources such as air, food and water to enable the body to heal itself. Symptoms are seen as the body's attempt to heal disease and restore health and harmony. The symptoms are therefore not to be suppressed but should be encouraged in healthy individuals. Treatment might include diet, fasting, hydrotherapy (water therapy), massage, osteopathy, exercise and relaxation techniques.

**What to expect** The main aim of diagnosis is to find out how well your vital force is working. The naturopath will perform some of the usual medical checks, such as taking your pulse and blood pressure as well as checking your body structurally to see how it is working. Treatment is extremely flexible and many of the treatments are not therapies as such but measures that are designed to be incorporated into your daily lifestyle for improved health.

Wholefoods form the core of the naturopathic diet and food should be as close as possible to its natural state (that is, preferably raw or only lightly cooked, and not processed in any way). Such a diet is naturally rich in fibre, which can help control the symptoms of IBS. The naturopath will be on the lookout for food intolerances and allergies, and may recommend an elimination diet (see Chapter 5, pages 109–110) or even a fast. Fasting is said to rest the digestive system, detoxify the body and stimulate the metabolism so that healing can take place. It should never be undertaken without supervision. The naturopath may also recommend avoiding irritants like coffee, strong spices and alcohol.

Hydrotherapy may be used to help stimulate the body's vital force. This may include the use of hot and cold compresses, cold baths, hot baths, saunas and sitz baths, where you sit in alternate hot and cold water. This can be especially useful for alleviating constipation. The therapist may also give you advice on exercise and relaxation and may show you how to massage your bowel in a gentle way. If IBS is accompanied by depression or anxiety, the therapist may also provide psychotherapy.

# Eastern therapies
## Ayurvedic medicine
Ayurvedic medicine is a traditional Eastern medical system practised mainly in India and Sri Lanka, but becoming much

more widely used in the West. It involves the use of a whole range of measures – diet, detoxification, yoga-type exercise, herbs and meditation – designed to help the body stay in balance and improve physical and mental health. In Ayurvedic medicine, each patient is treated individually according to their constitution. According to this thinking, your constitution is governed by three vital energies called the three *doshas*. These are known by their Sanskrit names of *vatha*, *pitha* and *kapha*.

## Ayurveda and IBS

In Ayurvedic medicine, good digestion is considered the key to good health. Poor digestion produces *ama*, a toxin believed to lie at the root of illness. *Ama* appears as a white coating on the tongue but can also line the colon. It occurs when the metabolism is disturbed due to an imbalance of *agni* or fire. *Agni* affected by too much *kapha* can slow digestion, making you feel heavy and sluggish, while too much *vatha* can cause wind, cramps and alternating constipation and diarrhoea – precisely the symptoms of IBS in fact.

While little scientific research has been carried out into Ayurvedic medicine in the West, one study carried out in India looked at 169 patients treated with either conventional treatment, a compound of Ayurvedic herbs or a placebo. Disappointingly, perhaps, the Ayurvedic preparation improved symptoms in 64.9 per cent of patients compared to 78.3 using standard medical treatment and 32.7 using the placebo. Researchers concluded that Ayurvedic treatment was useful in cases where diarrhoea was a dominant symptom. However, standard treatment seemed to be more useful for pain.

**What to expect** Diagnosis takes place at the first consultation. The practitioner will take a full medical history and will also want to know about your health as a child, your parents' health and your current lifestyle, all of which are factors that can affect your constitution. The practitioner will also observe you to try to determine which dosha is dominant and carry out a physical examination.

Treatment will usually involve detoxification – by means of massage with herbal oils designed to eliminate toxins, steam baths, enemas or inhalations. Herbal laxatives are often used to treat constipation and IBS. The practitioner will also usually prescribe herbal remedies – usually blends of different herbs made up specially for you – which you mix with water and boil, together with advice on exercise such as yoga and diet. There is no one healthy diet in Ayurveda, just a diet that is right for your constitution.

## Traditional Chinese medicine (TCM)

Like Ayurveda, Chinese medicine is a complete system of medicine which includes acupuncture, acupressure, Chinese herbalism, moxibustion (the use of burning herbs), massage, diet and physical exercise such as t'ai chi.

The aim of all these therapies is to balance the flow of *chi*, the body's vital force, upon which good health is said to depend. *Chi* flows around the body in invisible channels known as meridians, each of which is named after an organ or after a body function. When *chi* flows freely, the body is said to be balanced and healthy, but if *chi* becomes blocked, stagnated or weakened, this can result in physical, mental or emotional ill health.

## Acupuncture, acupressure and shiatsu

In acupuncture, needles are used to stimulate points located along the meridians to restore harmony and correct unbalanced *chi*. Acupressure and shiatsu involves stimulating the same points, only using pressure from the fingertips rather than needles, and massaging along the route of a meridian is meant to help balance the body's energies. Acupuncture has been used to help treat a number of gastrointestinal conditions including IBS and, although there have been few specific controlled trials, studies have shown that it can affect gut motility, nerve chemicals and hormones in the gut. It can also help raise the pain threshold. One, admittedly small, study of just seven patients showed a significant improvement in wellbeing and easing of bloating. A German study, comparing acupuncture with psychotherapy and drug treatment, found that acupuncture had a 31 per cent long-term success rate in controlling symptoms, although it was not as successful as psychotherapy which improved symptoms by 74 per cent.

Many people worry that acupuncture will be painful, but patients usually report that they cannot feel the needles at all, or that they feel a slight tingling sensation.

## Chinese herbal medicine

Chinese herbal medicine involves using mixtures of Chinese herbs made up into teas or decoctions to treat and prevent disease. The Chinese approach places an emphasis on prescribing herbs for you as an individual, although there are some standard compounds. Again, there have been few scientific trials to test how well it really works. However, in one randomized controlled trial carried out in Australia, in which

Chinese herbal preparations were tested against a placebo, the Chinese herbal treatments were significantly more effective, both in reducing symptoms of IBS and improving quality of life. Patients who did best over the long term were those whose treatment was individually prescribed for them.

**Caution** Herbs are prescribed to take into account all of the symptoms you are suffering from. Some Chinese herbs may not be safe for unsupervised use, and there have been some reports of problems with reactions to herbs which can affect the liver. For this reason, if you do decide to try this kind of treatment, it is vital to find a qualified practitioner who is registered with the Register of Chinese Herbal Medicine. It is also important to have regular blood checks to ensure your bone marrow, kidneys and liver are not being adversely affected by treatment. If you feel unwell, nauseous or develop diarrhoea or flu-like symptoms while taking Chinese herbs, stop taking them immediately and consult your practitioner.

**What to expect** Accurate diagnosis is the foundation for TCM, acupuncture and acupressure and Chinese herbal medicine, therefore, the practitioner will spend a long time examining you using the four traditional types of examination: looking, listening and smelling, asking and touching. The practitioner will observe your appearance and posture and, importantly, will specifically examine the colour of your complexion, your eyes and your tongue for signs of blocked *chi* or disharmony. They will also listen to your pattern of breathing and note the tone of your voice. Your body odour also gives clues as to your state of health. For example, a scorched smell reminiscent of freshly ironed

# USING COMPLEMENTARY THERAPIES

○ Remember that complementary therapies are meant to be used in addition to orthodox treatments not to replace them.

○ Find out as much as you can about a therapy before consulting a practitioner. Look at advantages and disadvantages, risks, side-effects, what improvements you can expect from treatment and how long treatment should take. Ask your doctor or check the Internet or medical journals.

○ Talk to people with IBS who have used complementary therapies. However, bear in mind that what works for them may not necessarily work for you.

○ Check out your practitioner carefully. See that he or she is registered with an appropriate professional body. Inspect the premises to make sure that they are clean and well-run.

○ If you don't like the person, no matter how illogical this is, go with your instinct and find someone else.

○ Ask the practitioner how many treatments you are likely to need. Beware of anyone who tries to sign you up for unlimited treatments.

○ Do not give up your conventional medication or treatment without the advice of your doctor.

○ Ensure that your orthodox doctor and complementary therapist are informed about any preparations you are taking, as some complementary treatments can interact with conventional medications and vice versa.

clothes is said to indicate an imbalance in 'fire', one of the four elements in Chinese medicine. The practitioner will ask you questions about yourself, your lifestyle, your general health and your relationships. He or she will also ask about any pain you are experiencing, as well as eating, sleeping and bowel habits. Finally, he or she might palpate your body and take your pulses. In Chinese medicine there are six pulses – three on each wrist – rather than the one of conventional Western medicine. The practitioner can test for up to 28 different qualities of pulse which indicate the state of your body's *chi*.

Once a diagnosis has been reached, the practitioner will prescribe herbs and/or acupuncture or acupressure, plus a number of other measures such as exercise or food, which are designed to help restore the balance of your body.

The exact course of treatment is tailored to you and your symptoms, so no two people with IBS will have the exact same course of treatment.

## The future for complementary therapies

As complementary treatments continue to rise in popularity, many orthodox practitioners are beginning to lose their scepticism and are even recommending complementary therapies to patients. With this increased medical interest, some complementary therapies are becoming the subject of mainstream scientific studies. It is increasingly likely in future that some of the boundaries between orthodox and complementary treatments will disappear even further. In the meantime, however, keep an open mind and make sure you are as well-informed as possible about any therapy you try – complementary or otherwise.

# 5 The role of food in IBS

Most people with IBS are aware that what and how they eat can have an effect on their symptoms. The wrong food choices can result in hours of discomfort and bloating, and frequent visits to the toilet or days of constipation. By making sure that you eat a healthy, nutritious diet and trying to steer clear of foods which aggravate symptoms, you can do a great deal to improve the quality of your daily life and prevent flare-ups.

In this chapter you will find the information and advice you need to take control of your diet and eating habits. It explains in detail how it is possible for food and drink to affect IBS and examines the various reasons why certain foods and drinks may trigger symptoms such as diarrhoea and constipation, bloating, pain and wind. Most important of all it gives practical advice on how you can modify your diet and eating habits to help improve any symptoms you might experience and reduce flare-ups.

# Improving your overall diet

Whatever the part played by food in provoking your particular symptoms, making sure you eat a healthy, nutritious diet will help you stay in better health and give you the energy you need to cope with your condition. It may also prevent symptoms from flaring up.

There's no one diet or food that suits everyone with IBS, so planning your diet will be a journey of discovery as you experiment to find out what you can and cannot eat. However, nutritionists and dieticians are now virtually unanimous in what they consider to be the optimum diet for health and wellbeing. If you make this the basis of your menu planning, within the constraints of your irritable bowel, you will feel more energetic and healthier.

By and large, food should be consumed as fresh as possible and as close to its natural state as possible – that is either raw, if you can tolerate it, or lightly steamed or grilled. Processed foods should be kept to a minimum since they are low in nutrients and may contain hidden ingredients that trigger symptoms in those with food sensitivity. You should get used to reading labels to check for ingredients such as modified starch, egg or food additives which may aggravate your IBS.

The easiest way to consume a balanced diet is to think of your food intake in terms of a plate containing portions of different kinds of food, such as starchy foods, proteins and vegetables. The relevant sections below will tell you what proportion of each food group your plate should contain. A certain amount of trial and error will probably be necessary to find the diet that best suits you within these guidelines.

## Starchy foods (carbohydrate)

The main portion on your plate should be starchy foods such as potatoes, wholegrain cereals, breads, pasta, rice and oats. These are low in fat, high in fibre and rich in complex carbohydrates, which are slowly digested and help sustain energy levels.

### Modifying your diet

You may find you can tolerate many starchy foods quite well. However, some starchy foods can provoke symptoms. For example, some people with IBS may be sensitive to gluten, a protein found in wheat, oats, barley and rye (see pages 111–112). If this applies to you, you may find you tolerate rice better (brown rice noodles, rice cakes), maize (corn) or buckwheat, millet, tapioca and sago. Yams, potatoes and sweet potatoes are usually fairly well tolerated as well. If you are sensitive to gluten watch out for hidden starch in processed foods (see pages 111–112).

## Fruit and vegetables

The next biggest portion on your plate should be fruit and vegetables, which are low in fat, high in fibre and rich in vitamins and minerals. Fruit and vegetables also contain other plant chemicals (phytochemicals), which doctors increasingly believe are important in preventing many of the diseases of Western civilization, such as heart disease, diabetes, cancer and degenerative diseases of ageing.

## Modifying your diet

Some fruits and vegetables can trigger wind and diarrhoea, especially when eaten raw. Foods which are particularly wind-inducing include onions, leeks, garlic, shallots, Brussels sprouts, cabbage, cauliflower, broccoli, peas and beans, Jerusalem artichokes, the herb fennel and asafoetida, used in Indian cooking. Some fresh fruits may also be poorly tolerated, possibly because of a sensitivity to fructose, fruit sugar. Dried fruits like apricots, raisins and figs can also be problematic for the same reason in some sufferers.

Cooking can sometimes make fruit and vegetables more digestible, or try eating canned varieties. True, cooking does destroy vitamin C, one of the most valuable antioxidants (substances that zap free radicals – harmful molecules thought to lie behind diseases such as cancer, diabetes and heart disease). However, some nutrients are better absorbed when food is cooked. For example, the antioxidant vitamin beta carotene is best absorbed from carrots when they are cooked with a little fat.

If you are worried about getting enough vitamin C, you could consider taking a supplement. Another supplement that may be worth considering is the enzyme alpha-galactosidase – available from health food shops and mail order nutrient companies – which breaks down indigestible starches and may reduce wind.

# Protein foods

The third largest portion on your plate should consist of protein: meat, fish, poultry or plant-based sources of protein such as peas, beans, lentils, nuts and seeds. As well as protein, these foods contain vitamins, iron and zinc.

## Modifying your diet

The hard, saturated fat found in animal products is particularly difficult to digest and may irritate the gut, so select lean cuts of meat and poultry without skin, and grill, steam or stir-fry rather than deep-frying or roasting. Some people with IBS also find that red meat triggers symptoms, so – unless you are vegetarian – you may find it better to get most of your protein from white meat and fish.

Pulses are a good source of protein and low in fat. However, some people with IBS find that they worsen symptoms such as wind and bloating. Careful attention to the preparation of pulses can help. Pulses should be soaked for six to eight hours or left to soak overnight, and soya beans should be soaked for one to two days, changing the water daily. Drain and rinse well before cooking.

Some pulses – notably red kidney beans, borlotti, aduki and black beans – contain an enzyme that can cause stomach upsets in anyone, not just people with IBS. When you cook them, you should first bring them to the boil and simmer for a full ten minutes before draining, discarding the cooking water, adding fresh water and cooking as usual.

Some people find they can tolerate certain pulses and not others. Some trial and error may be necessary to find ones that suit you.

# Milk and dairy foods

The next largest portion of food on your plate should be milk and dairy foods, such as yogurt, cheese and milk. These are an important food group for providing protein, calcium and other vitamins.

## Modifying your diet

Dairy foods can be particular offenders in triggering symptoms of IBS, possibly because of lactose intolerance (see pages 110–111). Yogurt is often better tolerated because the lactose is broken down and live yogurt is also beneficial as a source of *Lactobacillus acidophilus*, a type of bacterium which helps maintain levels of healthy bacteria in the bowel.

# Fatty, sugary foods

The smallest portion on the plate should be fatty, sugary foods. This includes biscuits, doughnuts, crisps, snacks, ice cream, mayonnaise, bottled sauces, honey, sweets, chocolate and sweet drinks, which are high in calories but low in nutrients.

## Modifying your diet

Fatty sugary foods are best avoided altogether or kept strictly for the occasional treat, for those who do and those who don't suffer from IBS. However, these foods can contain a double whammy for people with IBS, as sugar and fat can make symptoms worse. These foods may also contain ingredients such as wheat, milk and yeast, which may be a source of sensitivity in some sufferers.

# Good fats and bad fats

Hard saturated fats found in meat and animal products, such as butter and cheese, and transfats found in processed foods are hard to digest and can irritate the bowel. Many IBS sufferers find that a heavy, rich meal triggers diarrhoea.

The best kinds of fats for health – and possibly also for your bowel – are the monounsaturated kind found in olive oil and avocado, sesame and walnut oil. These fats seem to help regulate gut activity and prevent the rapid bowel transit which leads to diarrhoea.

You should also try to boost your intake of essential fatty acids or EFAs (sometimes known as vitamin F). These are a group of unsaturated fats which are found particularly in nuts, seeds, vegetables and oily fish. The two main EFAs are omega-3 and omega-6.

## SOURCES OF EFAS

**Omega-3:**
- Salmon
- Swordfish
- Herring
- Mackerel
- Tuna
- Hemp seeds
- Flax seeds
- Pumpkin seeds

**Omega-6:**
- Vegetables
- Hemp seeds
- Sunflower seeds
- Pumpkin seeds
- Sesame seeds
- Evening primrose oil
- Borage (starflower) oil

The balance between omega-6 and omega-3 is important and nutritional experts recommend twice as much omega-6 as omega-3. To ensure you get the correct balance:

❑ Use a cold-pressed, ready-blended omega-6/omega-3 oil mix (available from health food and whole food stores) on vegetables and salads.

❑ Take an EFA supplement.

❑ Sprinkle nuts and seeds over salads or breakfast cereals.

A high carbohydrate consumption increases the need for unsaturated fats. These fats, unlike saturated fats, actually help the body burn fat, which is a bonus if you are trying to control your weight.

## The fibre factor

Fibre, the indigestible part of plants, fruits, seeds and nuts, is an important part of a healthy diet. Fibre works by absorbing water as it passes through your digestive system, producing a stool that is soft, bulky and easy to pass without strain. Insufficient leads to smaller, drier stools, which means that the walls of the gut have to contract more forcefully to push them through, and constipation results.

Unfortunately, the processed, highly refined diet many people eat today is extremely low in fibre. In fact, research suggests that most of us fall far short of the recommended daily intake of fibre. Many health experts attribute the rise of diseases such as bowel and other cancers and a number of digestive disorders to this lack of fibre.

The role of fibre in IBS is complicated and controversial. For a long time, a low-fibre diet was recommended for IBS sufferers. Then, in the 1970s, with new findings on the benefits of fibre,

## SOURCES OF FIBRE

**Soluble:**

○ Apples

○ Barley

○ Brown rice

○ Citrus fruits

○ Dried fruits e.g. currants, figs, raisins

○ Oats

○ Psyllium seed

○ Pulses e.g. lentils, dried beans, peas

○ Rice

○ Soya beans

○ Squash

**Insoluble:**

○ Bran

○ Breakfast cereals with added bran

○ Flax seed

○ Peppers

○ Potatoes

○ Strawberries

○ Wholemeal bread and pasta

a high-fibre diet was recommended. More recently still, however, doctors have begun to question whether certain types of fibre may actually aggravate symptoms for some sufferers, and they are again recommending a low-fibre diet. True, many people with IBS, especially those in whom constipation is a dominant symptom, find that eating a fibre-rich diet helps. However, others, particularly those in whom diarrhoea is a dominant symptom, can find that fibre makes their symptoms worse. Once again, it's simply a question of trial and error to see what suits you.

## Types of fibre

For many of us, the term fibre conjures up an image of a handful of bran, but in fact bran is just one kind of fibre. Basically, fibre is the indigestible part of plants, fruit and vegetables and it is not just one substance but a whole family of different ones. The husk on a grain of wheat is fibre (when milled it forms wheat bran), so is the skin on an apple. But fibre is also what gives porridge or a stew containing barley a gluey consistency, and it's also the substance that gives jams and preserves their sticky, gelatinous quality.

The fibre in the husks surrounding grains and the skin of certain vegetables and fruit is known as insoluble fibre, because it doesn't dissolve in water. Soluble fibre, on the other hand, does dissolve in water, and is found in oats, barley, pulses and dried fruits.

Because it makes stools bulkier, fibre can help prevent the colon from overcontracting and going into spasm, and can ease both constipation and diarrhoea.

Soluble fibre seems to be far better tolerated and more beneficial than insoluble fibre, which can be hard to digest. In particular, sprinkling extra fibre such as wheat bran on food is generally not advisable because it often exacerbates symptoms, especially in those IBS sufferers who are sensitive to gluten, a type of protein found in wheat.

## Fibre frenzy

Before the 1970s, most conventional dieticians and nutritionists dismissed dietary fibre as unimportant. But then research emerged showing that rural Africans who were eating a high-fibre diet were less likely to develop Western diseases such as bowel and other cancers, diverticulosis, gallstones, haemorrhoids and constipation, and were less likely to be overweight than people eating a typical refined Western diet. A slew of popular books and articles appeared extolling the benefits of fibre, sales of wheat bran soared and bran was added to everything from breakfast cereals to drinks. Today, while the importance of dietary fibre is undisputed, doctors and scientists are coming to a more sophisticated understanding of the types of fibre that are most beneficial. There's less emphasis on adding bran to food and more on taking fibre in the way nature intended – that is wrapped up in fruit, vegetables, nuts, seeds and grains.

## Introducing more fibre into your diet

The best way to get more fibre is to eat a diet rich in fruit, vegetables and wholegrain cereals, rather than sprinkling bran over your food. If you have been used to consuming a highly refined diet, you may find that when you first start eating a more fibrous diet, wind and bloating get worse. Take it slowly and give your digestive system time to get used to your new eating habits. You will probably find that as your body adjusts, symptoms will dwindle. This can take several weeks, so be patient and persevere.

Many people find that, after a few weeks on a diet that is high in fibre, bowel movements become more regular and other symptoms diminish. If they don't, you may need to examine your diet more closely to see whether fibre is the culprit, or whether it is some other aspect of your diet. If you decide fibre is to blame, you may want to try reducing it until you find the level that you can tolerate. Alternatively, you could ask your doctor about fibre supplements. The most useful kind are those based on psyllium, a type of soluble fibre. As with so much to do with IBS, it's very much a question of being patient until you find the regimen that suits you best.

# The importance of water

It's vital to increase your water intake when you eat a high-fibre diet, since water is absorbed by fibre and helps move it through the gut. Water is also particularly important if diarrhoea is a dominant symptom of your IBS, to avoid dehydration. Aim to drink 2–2.5 litres (3½–4½ pints) a day, and more when you exercise. This may sound a lot, but if you have a glass or bottle of water by you and take regular sips throughout the day you will find it is not as difficult as it appears. Water used in tea and coffee does not count, because caffeine is a diuretic and causes water loss from the body. If you find plain water boring, perk it up by adding a slice or two of orange or lime, some grated fresh root ginger or a sprig of mint.

## Drinks

Caffeine, which is found in tea, coffee, hot chocolate, colas, some soft drinks, 'alcopops' and some medications, can affect the motility of the gut. Caffeine is a stimulant which can lead to anxiety and nervousness (both of which can exacerbate IBS) and can also provoke diarrhoea, wind and a rumbling stomach.

Caffeine is also associated with symptoms such as tension headaches, migraine and irritable bladder, which as we've seen can also be more common in people with IBS. All good reasons to cut down on caffeine or cut it out altogether and substitute water and herbal teas.

Conversely, however, tea has been linked with an increased tendency to constipation, which may be problematic if constipation is a dominant symptom.

It's also worth bearing in mind that hot drinks can trigger peristaltic waves. If you notice that this is a factor for you, you may want to cut down on hot drinks. Many experts think that drinking beverages at body temperature is best.

A high alcohol consumption can deplete nutrients and disturb the body's metabolism of essential fatty acids. Gassy alcoholic drinks, such as beer and lager, are particular culprits when it comes to bloating and wind, partly because they contain gas and partly perhaps because of the additives used to preserve them. Wines and certain spirits can aggravate diarrhoea, especially in people who are sensitive to yeast or grains. In any case, moderating your alcohol intake is beneficial for health and women should consume no more than one to two units a day and men no more than three or four. A unit is equivalent to half a pint of beer or lager, a small glass of wine or a pub measure of spirits.

# Eating patterns and habits

Because stress plays such an important part in IBS, how you eat can be important as well as what you eat. Irregular or hurried meals or meals eaten in tense or uncomfortable conditions can aggravate wind, bloating and abdominal discomfort. Skipping meals can lead to a slowdown in the secretion of digestive enzymes. Large, heavy meals can overload your gut, leading to abdominal discomfort and diarrhoea. Eating too fast and talking while you eat can exacerbate bloating and discomfort, because they encourage you to swallow air.

When you eat, it is important to relax and give yourself time to enjoy your food. Eating at your desk or grabbing a quick snack as you do something else is stressful and encourages the bowel to contract, causing abdominal pain. It's also more likely to induce wind, especially if you swallow your food before you have chewed it properly. Many people with IBS find that eating little and often is easier on their digestive system than three heavy meals. Try having three smallish meals a day, plus two or three light nutritious snacks. When eating, avoid bolting your food and concentrate on chewing slowly and thoroughly. Try to avoid skipping meals. If you think it's going to be difficult to eat, perhaps because of a meeting or travel, make sure that you take a light snack or two with you.

## Food sensitivity

There is still a great deal of controversy in the medical profession about the role of food sensitivity in IBS. The issue is a tangled one. A number of studies have been conducted into the relationship between food and IBS, and while several have suggested that foods are a problem, none have proved conclusively that food allergy or intolerance are definite factors. Having said this, practically everyone with IBS can point to at least one or two foods that don't agree with them, although the exact reason for this is still up for debate.

# Food allergy or food intolerance?

Before discussing how to find out if food is a factor for you, it's important to make a distinction between food allergy – sometimes known as immediate food sensitivity – and food intolerance, or delayed food hypersensitivity.

## Food allergy

Food allergy, in the strict sense of the term, is fairly rare. It involves the immune system, the body's defence mechanism. When exposed to a certain food, the body wrongly reacts as if it were being attacked and produces antibodies to fight off the invader, just as it would from an onslaught by a virus or bacterium. Common foods that cause an allergy are known as allergens, and include milk, wheat, shellfish, eggs, soya, peanuts, walnuts, pecans and citrus fruit.

Only a small amount of food is needed to trigger a reaction (sometimes just handling a plate on which there is a portion of the offending food is enough) and symptoms usually come on immediately. Many experts term this type of reaction immediate food hypersensitivity.

It is thought that people who react to food in this way have a leaky gut, which allows molecules of semi-digested food to enter the bloodstream, triggering the release of inflammatory chemicals from the immune system.

There are several tests that can be used to find our whether or not you have a food allergy. These include skin prick testing, when a drop of a suspected allergen is scratched into the skin to see if it provokes a reaction, and a variety of blood tests designed to measure levels of antibodies. None of these tests is foolproof, however.

## Food intolerance

The other type of food sensitivity is food intolerance, also known as delayed food hypersensitivity or masked food allergy. In this type of reaction, symptoms develop some time after the offending food is consumed – anything from six to twenty-four hours but sometimes even longer – and the effects can go on for hours or days.

The mechanism underlying this type of food sensitivity remains a mystery. However, there are several clues that can help you pinpoint if this is your problem:

❑ Triggers tend to be common foods you eat frequently and in relatively large quantities.

❑ Symptoms come and go: food you can eat with no problems one day may upset you on another occasion. Sometimes foods you have eaten without a problem for years can trigger a reaction.

❑ Often there is a variety of symptoms rather than one definitive reaction. These can include itching, headaches, fatigue, fluid retention, muscle and joint aches and pains, flushes, sweats, diarrhoea, constipation, wind and indigestion.

❑ Trigger foods are often foods you like a lot or even crave. In fact, when you first eliminate them you may feel worse rather than better.

# Detecting food sensitivity

Keeping a food diary (see page 112), will help you identify patterns of symptoms and the foods they are linked with. However, by far the best way to identify whether food sensitivity is a problem for you is to go on an exclusion or elimination diet in which you systematically leave out foods that cause problems and then reintroduce them one by one to see whether they provoke symptoms.

# Exclusion diets

Going on an exclusion diet is stressful and time-consuming. Each food must be excluded for up to three weeks to detect if it is problematic, and you have to be very strict as only half excluding something will make results impossible to interpret. Furthermore if, as is common, several foods are culprits, it can take some time to check them all.

For these reasons, although it is possible to go it alone, an exclusion diet is far better followed under the supervision of a doctor, dietician or nutritional therapist, who can support you and help you interpret results.

## Points to bear in mind

**Be prepared** Go shopping for foods that you are allowed to eat and clear your fridge and cupboards of forbidden foods so you won't be tempted.

**Pick your time** Avoid Christmas and other festivals, birthdays or holidays. These can be stressful enough in themselves and it may be virtually impossible to stick to the diet. Many people find it best to start over a weekend or when they have a few days off so that they have time and easy access to permitted foods.

**Have patience** It can take anything from a couple of days to two or three weeks before an improvement is felt and initially symptoms may actually worsen when you first exclude a food. This aggravation is considered to be a good sign because it indicates that food sensitivity is indeed a problem.

**Get nutrient wise** Before starting to exclude foods from your diet, make sure you are getting all the nutrients you need. This can be achieved by taking a supplement. Check the packet carefully since some contain substances to which you may be sensitive, such as yeast or starch. If in doubt, consult a nutritional therapist.

**Don't go on indefinitely** Remember an exclusion diet is intended to diagnose food sensitivity, not to be continued indefinitely. Indeed if you stay on it for a long time, you could become seriously short of nutrients.

**Check symptoms** After three weeks of leaving out suspect foods, reintroduce a normal size portion of the food into your diet, one food at a time, and use your diary to record symptoms. You'll need to allow up to 36 hours for an adverse reaction to appear. If a reaction does occur, leave out the offending food and wait for symptoms to abate before reintroducing another food, otherwise the results could become confused.

# Common food and drink triggers

## Dairy products

Milk, cheese, ice cream and chocolate are common culprits. In some cases, this may be due to an inability to tolerate or process lactose, or milk sugar, due to an underlying deficiency of the digestive enzyme lactase. Processed foods that may contain cows' milk include bread, cakes, biscuits, malt drinks, puddings, ice cream, soups and sauces. Many homoeopathic remedies are in the form of pills made of milk sugar. If lactose is a problem for you, your homoeopathic practitioner will usually be able to prescribe the remedy in a different form, such as a tincture. Check processed food labels for skimmed milk powder, non-fat milk solids, caseine, whey lactalbumen. Some people find goats' and sheep's milk are better tolerated than cows' milk.

## Eggs

Although eggs are commonly reputed to be 'binding', this is a myth and if you are sensitive to them they can cause diarrhoea. You may be sensitive to either yolk or white, or both. Watch out for foods such as cakes, biscuits, puddings, batter, egg noodles, egg pasta, mayonnaise and many other processed foods since these may contain hidden egg. It's important to check labels.

## Sugar and artificial sweeteners

Sugar doesn't appear to be a major culprit in IBS. However, some people can be sensitive to certain sorts of sugar such as glucose and fruit sugar. Sorbitol, an artificial sweetener found in many diet foods and drinks and even in some drugs and medicines, can trigger diarrhoea, so check labels.

## Wheat, oats, barley and rye

All these contain gluten. If you are sensitive to wheat you may be able to tolerate oats, barley and rye better, but not always. Check processed food labels carefully. Modified starch, wheat, wheat starch, edible starch, cereal filler, cereal binder and cereal protein may all contain wheat and should be avoided.

Corn (maize or sweetcorn) does not contain gluten and is sometimes better tolerated by those suffering from IBS. However it too can be a source of sensitivity. Many foods contain hidden corn in the form of edible starch or corn syrup. All kinds of food, including maize oil and vegetable oils and margarines, baking powders, cakes, biscuits, sauces, puddings and even some baked beans can also be sources of corn.

## KEEPING A FOOD DIARY

Keeping a food diary is similar to keeping a trigger diary as outlined in Chapter 2, page 34. Here are some reminders:

○ Use a soft-backed notebook or diary small enough to carry with you when you go out.

○ Record what you eat and drink as you go along rather than later in the day, since it's easy to forget.

○ Record what you ate and when in as much detail as possible – include how the food was cooked, how much you ate and any dressings or condiments used.

○ Include the circumstances in which you ate or drank, for example who you were with, what you were doing and how you felt (relaxed or tense), as all of these can affect digestion.

○ If you are a woman, include the stage of your menstrual cycle.

○ Record IBS symptoms: your bowel movements, the consistency of your stools, whether mucus is present, abdominal discomfort or pain and/or bloating.

Over a period of four to six weeks you may begin to notice a distinct pattern emerging, which you can use to moderate your diet.

## Yeast

Yeast is found in many foods and in most alcoholic drinks (apart from gin, vodka and other spirits such as plum brandy which are filtered rather than fermented). Obviously a major source of yeast is any bread that has been proved, since yeast is used to make the bread rise. Matzos, chapattis, puris, parathas and Mediterranean and Middle Eastern flat breads may be better tolerated, provided you are not sensitive to grains.

You also need to be on the lookout for products coated in breadcrumbs, such as fish cakes, fish fingers, chicken goujons and potato croquettes. Other foods that may cause problems include yeast extract, certain vitamin supplements (especially those containing vitamin B), crisps and other savoury snacks, packet soups, stock cubes and gravies.

Natural yeasts are present in vinegar and pickled foods, over-ripe or mouldy fruits, fruit juices, grapes and mushrooms. A reaction to yeast can be worsened by consuming sugar and refined starches which encourage the growth of yeast.

# Eating a balanced diet

Once you have some idea of the foods that affect you, you should find you feel better if you eliminate them from your diet. Some IBS sufferers find that simply reducing their intake of a particular food or foods can help; others find that they have to eliminate them completely to get relief.

The best diet for all-round good health is a balanced diet, so if you do decide to eliminate a food, it's important to make sure that a nutritious alternative introduced, otherwise you may find that you are lacking essential nutrients. If you appear to be sensitive to several different kinds of food or are finding it difficult to modify your diet, seek the advice of a doctor, dietician or nutritionist who can help you plan a balanced, nutritious diet.

After six months to a year you may find you can introduce offending foods again, a little at a time. If they don't cause renewed symptoms you may be able to include small quantities in your diet, without it causing problems. For example, you may be able to have a dash of milk in your tea or eat a small piece of cheese, although you'll probably need to keep offending foods to a minimum to prevent troublesome symptoms appearing again.

## Spices and herbs

Many people with IBS find that cuisines and dishes that use a lot of spices and herbs can trigger symptoms. These include Indian, Mexican, Thai and Afro-Caribbean. If you enjoy foods from these cuisines, you will probably find that you can tolerate certain herbs and spices better than others – hot spices like chilli and capsicum, for example, frequently spark off symptoms. With a bit of experimentation and careful choices you will usually find a few dishes you can eat. Herbs such as fennel, sunflower and poppy can cause wind, while asafoetida, a ground herb used in Indian cooking, can cause smelly wind.

## A candida connection?

Some writers on IBS believe that candidiasis, caused by an excess of *Candida albicans*, a yeast found naturally in the gut, can trigger the condition. Factors that can encourage candida include lowered immunity, long-term or repeated courses of antibiotics, diabetes, the contraceptive pill, pregnancy and dietary deficiencies.

As well as IBS, there may be a range of other symptoms of candidiasis, including oral or vaginal thrush, fatigue, irritability, headaches, joint and muscle pains, rashes, fungal infections such as athlete's foot, vaginal and/or anal itching recurrent cystitis and food cravings. Symptoms may be worsened by foods and drugs containing yeast or sugar, and by low or damp places which may contain moulds. Candidiasis can be treated with high doses of anti-fungal drugs and an anti-candida diet, which bans refined carbohydrates and yeast-containing foods and drinks, and includes foods containing natural anti-fungal ingredients such as garlic, olive oil and fresh green leafy vegetables.

The candida connection is still extremely controversial, however, among orthodox experts. If you think you might be affected, especially if diarrhoea and bloating are dominant symptoms of your IBS, it may be worth asking your doctor to prescribe an anti-fungal treatment and trying an anti-candida diet. You may need to continue for twelve weeks, although most people notice an improvement within two to six weeks. If after three months you haven't seen an improvement, the chances are that candida is not the root of your problem.

# Dealing with specific symptoms

The following summarizes the dietary recommendations outlined in this chapter for specific IBS symptoms.

## Diarrhoea

❑ Check for food sensitivity: milk, wheat and alcohol may be particular culprits

❑ Cut down on or cut out coffee and caffeinated drinks

- ❑ Don't sprinkle bran on your food – soluble fibre found in fruit and vegetables is usually better tolerated
- ❑ Limit consumption of hot, spicy foods
- ❑ Limit fatty foods
- ❑ Avoid pulses and beans if they cause problems
- ❑ Include olive oil in your diet
- ❑ Eat little and often. Avoid skipping meals
- ❑ Drink plenty of plain water – at least six to eight glasses (2.5 litres/4½ pints) a day
- ❑ Avoid sorbitol, an artificial sweetener found in many diet foods and drinks, and chewing gum
- ❑ Watch out for certain fruits, especially dried fruits like apricots and figs

## Constipation

- ❑ Check for food sensitivity: wheat and grains may be culprits and less often milk and dairy products
- ❑ Step up your intake of fibre. Base your diet around whole grains, starchy foods, fresh fruit and vegetables
- ❑ You may find sprinkling extra bran on your food is helpful, although it is generally better to take your fibre in the way nature intended, i.e. in fruit and vegetables
- ❑ Cut down on tea. Substitute herbal teas and water
- ❑ Drink plenty of fluids – at least six to eight glasses of water a day (2.5 litres/4½ pints)
- ❑ Eat little and often. Avoid skipping meals

## Wind and bloating

- ❑ Check for food sensitivity: milk, wheat, other grains and yeast can be particular culprits

- Certain fruits, especially dried fruits such as apricots, raisins and figs may cause problems
- Take your time over your meals and eat slowly, chewing food well.
- Avoid carbonated soft drinks and fizzy alcoholic drinks such as beer and lager
- Check if wine is a problem: it may be if you are sensitive to yeast
- Soak and cook pulses thoroughly. If this doesn't help, keep them to a minimum
- Beer, white wine and fruit juices can cause smelly gas in some people. If this applies to you, avoid them
- Steer clear of vegetables from the cabbage family such as broccoli, cabbage and Brussels sprouts
- Avoid garlic, onions, leeks and other gas-producing foods
- Avoid sorbitol, an artificial sweetener found in diet foods and drinks, and chewing gum
- Avoid herbs and spices such as fennel, sunflower, poppy and asafoetida

# Sample menus

## Menu for diarrhoea-dominant IBS

### Breakfast

Rice cereal with soya milk and blueberries

Rooibos tea (a nourishing, caffeine-free South African tea, which is also low in tannin) with soya milk if dairy milk not tolerated

Orange juice

### Snack

Millet and cranberry flapjacks

Water

**Lunch**

Hummus with flat bread, grilled asparagus salad (page 184)

Banana, nuts or any fruit you can tolerate

**Snack**

Rice cakes

Peppermint tea

**Supper**

Sea bass with fennel (page 158)

Melon ice cream (page 213)

Camomile tea

# Menu for constipation-dominant IBS
**Breakfast**

Mighty muesli (page 162)

Orange juice

Herbal tea or coffee substitute

**Snack**

Slice wholemeal bread with mashed banana

Peppermint tea

**Lunch**

Grilled chicken, butternut squash and wilted spinach salad (page 106)

Fruit

**Snack**

Piece of fruit

Peppermint tea

**Supper**

Peperonata with wholemeal noodles and green salad (page 194)

Stuffed figs (page 164)

Camomile tea

# 6 Exclusion recipes

This chapter shows how easy it is to concoct delicious, nutrient-rich meals based around fresh ingredients – even if you have to leave out certain foods. It can be difficult to find interesting and nutritious recipes if you are excluding common ingredients, so the recipes here are designed to exclude common foods that can provoke sensitivity, and provide exciting ideas for healthy dishes to tempt your and your family's taste buds.

Here you will find ideas for every kind of meal, from soups and main dishes to salads, snacks and puddings. Each recipe has been analysed and you can use this to plan your menus. Once you've got used to cooking in this way, you can adapt the recipes in this and the next chapter to avoid foods that upset your digestive system.

# Soups and starters

## Pea and mint soup

alcohol free ✓ I citrus free ✓ I dairy free ✗ I gluten free ✓ I wheat free ✓

**Serves 6**
**Preparation time: 5–10 minutes**
**Cooking time: 30–35 minutes**

**Per serving**
Energy 140 kcals/593 kJ I Protein 7 g I Carbohydrate 20 g I Fat 5 g
Fibre 7 g

25 g (1 oz) butter or margarine
1 small onion, chopped
500 g (1 lb) frozen green peas
¼ teaspoon sugar
1.2 litres (2 pints) Chicken Stock (see page 175)
4 tablespoons chopped mint
300 g (10 oz) potatoes, roughly chopped
150 ml (¼ pint) semi-skimmed milk
salt and white pepper

**1** Melt the butter or margarine in a saucepan, add the onion and cook over a moderate heat until soft but not coloured, stirring frequently.

**2** Add the peas, sugar and stock and 3 tablespoons of the chopped mint. Stir in white pepper to taste and bring the mixture to the boil. Add the potatoes, lower the heat and simmer, partially covered, for 20–25 minutes.

**3** Allow the mixture to cool slightly, then purée the mixture in batches in a food processor or blender until smooth. Return to a clean saucepan, season with salt, add the milk and stir well. Heat the soup gently without boiling. Serve in warmed soup plates or bowls, garnished with the remaining mint.

# Carrot and sage soup

alcohol free ✓ | citrus free ✓ | dairy free ✗ | gluten free ✓ | wheat free ✓

**Serves 6**
**Preparation time: 15 minutes**
**Cooking time: about 1 hour**

**Per serving**
Energy 90 kcals/373 kJ | Protein 1 g | Carbohydrate 13 g | Fat 4 g
Fibre 4 g

25 g (1 oz) butter
1 large onion, finely chopped
750 g (1½ lb) carrots, finely sliced
900 ml (1½ pints) vegetable stock
1 tablespoon chopped sage
salt and pepper
sage sprigs, to garnish

**1** Melt the butter in a large heavy-based pan, add the onion and
   fry gently until soft but not coloured, then add the carrots and
   stock and season with salt and pepper. Bring to the boil and
   simmer uncovered for about 30 minutes.

**2** Allow the soup to cool slightly, then purée the soup in a food
   processor or blender until smooth, then return to a clean pan
   and add the chopped sage. Return to the boil and simmer for
   another 15 minutes.

**3** Serve the soup garnished with sage sprigs.

# Red lentil soup

alcohol free ✓ | citrus free ✓ | dairy free ✓ | gluten free ✓ | wheat free ✓

**Serves 4**
**Preparation time: 10 minutes**
**Cooking time: about 30–35 minutes**

**Per serving**
Energy 220 kcals/938 kJ | Protein 16 g | Carbohydrate 40 g | Fat 1 g
Fibre 9 g

250 g (8 oz) split red lentils
1 leek, sliced
2 large carrots, sliced
1 celery stick, sliced
1 garlic clove, crushed (optional)
1 bay leaf
1.2 litres (2 pints) vegetable stock
½ teaspoon cayenne pepper
pepper

To Garnish:
very-low-fat natural yogurt

**1** Place all the ingredients for the soup in a large saucepan, bring
   to the boil, cover and simmer for 20–25 minutes or until the
   lentils and all the vegetables are tender.

**2** Allow the soup to cool slightly and remove the bay leaf. Purée
   the soup in batches in a food processor or blender until smooth.

**3** Return the soup to a clean saucepan, season with pepper, and
   heat through. To serve, transfer to warmed soup plates or bowls,
   garnishing each portion with a swirl of yogurt.

# Crab and rice soup

alcohol free ✓ I citrus free ✓ I dairy free ✓ I gluten free ✕ I wheat free ✕

**Serves 6**
**Preparation time: 15 minutes**
**Cooking time: 1¼ hours**

**Per serving**
Energy 334 kcals/1407 kJ I Protein 20 g I Carbohydrate 38 g I Fat 12 g
Fibre 2 g

500 g (1 lb) white crab meat
4 tablespoons olive oil
1 onion, chopped
250 g (8 oz) tomatoes, skinned and chopped
1 teaspoon paprika
1.8 litres (3 pints) boiling water
2 garlic cloves
2 parsley sprigs, leaves stripped from the stems
3 saffron threads
250 g (8 oz) long-grain white rice
salt
croûtons, to garnish (optional)

**1** Cut the crab meat into 1 cm (½ inch) pieces. Heat the oil in a heavy-based saucepan and sauté the crab meat until lightly browned. Add the onion and cook over a moderate heat for 5 minutes, stirring constantly. Add the tomatoes, paprika, ½ teaspoon salt and the boiling water. Cover the pan and cook over a low heat for about 45 minutes.

**2** Meanwhile, pound the garlic cloves in a mortar with a pinch of salt and the parsley sprigs. Add the saffron and 2 tablespoons of the simmering stock. Stir the mixture well.

**3** Add the rice and the garlic mixture to the saucepan. Simmer, partially covered, for 20 minutes, until the rice is tender. Turn off the heat and leave the soup to rest on the stove for 2–3 minutes. Stir and adjust the seasoning if necessary. Pour the soup into a heated tureen and serve hot with croûtons, if using.

# Hummus

alcohol free ✓  |  citrus free ✕  |  dairy free ✓  |  gluten free ✓  |  wheat free ✓

**Serves 6**
**Preparation time: 20 minutes, plus overnight soaking and chilling**
**Cooking time: 1–1½ hours**

**Per serving**
Energy 415 kcals/1730 kJ  |  Protein 18 g  |  Carbohydrate 22 g  |  Fat 29 g
Fibre 6 g

250 g (8 oz) dried chickpeas, soaked overnight, drained and rinsed
2–3 garlic cloves, crushed with a little salt
about 250 ml (8 fl oz) lemon juice
about 5 tablespoons tahini
salt

To Garnish:
extra virgin olive oil
paprika

**1** Cook the chickpeas in a large saucepan of boiling water until
soft: 1–1½ hours. Drain and reserve the cooking liquid. Purée the
chickpeas in a food processor or blender with a little of the
cooking liquid, then press through a sieve to remove the skins.

**2** Beat the garlic into the chickpea purée. Stir in the lemon juice
and tahini alternately, tasting to get the right balance of flavours.
Add a little more salt, if necessary, and more of the cooking
liquid to make a soft, creamy consistency. Spoon the purée into a
shallow dish, cover and leave in the refrigerator for several hours.

**3** Return the hummus to room temperature before serving. Make
swirls in the surface, then trickle over olive oil and sprinkle with
paprika. Serve with pitta bread or crudités.

# Guacamole

alcohol free ✓ | citrus free ✕ | dairy free ✓ | gluten free ✓ | wheat free ✓

**Serves 4–6**
**Preparation time: 15 minutes, plus chilling**

**Per serving**
Energy 195 kcals/805 kJ | Protein 3 g | Carbohydrate 3 g | Fat 19 g
Fibre 1 g

2 large ripe avocados
3 tablespoons lemon or lime juice
2 garlic cloves, crushed
40 g (1½ oz) spring onions, chopped
1–2 tablespoons chopped mild green chillies
125 g (4 oz) tomatoes, skinned, deseeded and chopped
salt and pepper
rind of 1 lime, cut into strips, to garnish

**1** Cut the avocados in half and remove the stones. Scoop out the
flesh into a bowl, add the lemon or lime juice and mash coarsely.

**2** Add the garlic, spring onions and chillies, and season to taste
with salt and pepper. Mix in the chopped tomatoes. Cover and
chill in the refrigerator for at least 1 hour.

**3** Garnish the guacamole with strips of lime rind and serve with
crudités, tortilla chips or crackers.

# Chilled stuffed artichokes

alcohol free ✓  I  citrus free ✕  I  dairy free ✓  I  gluten free ✓  I  wheat free ✓

**Serves 4**
**Preparation time: 20 minutes, plus chilling**
**Cooking time: about 35 minutes**

**Per serving**
Energy 217 kcals/909 kJ  I  Protein 13 g  I  Carbohydrate 32 g  I  Fat 5 g
Fibre 2 g

4 artichokes, stems trimmed and top third of leaves removed
1 tablespoon lemon juice

Gingered Vegetables:
3 carrots, cut into rounds
75 g (3 oz) cauliflower florets
75 g (3 oz) broccoli florets
2 small courgettes, cut into rounds
3.5 cm (1½ inch) piece root ginger, peeled and cut into strips

Sauce:
150 g (5 oz) tofu, drained and roughly chopped
4 tablespoons tomato purée
4 tablespoons horseradish sauce
2 teaspoons lemon juice
2 teaspoons white wine vinegar
½ teaspoon onion salt
½ teaspoon sugar
a few drops of Tabasco sauce
½ teaspoon grated lemon rind
pepper

1 Place the artichokes and lemon juice in a deep saucepan and add boiling water to cover. Cover and cook for 30 minutes, or until one of the artichoke leaves pulls off easily. Remove the artichokes from the pan, turn them upside down to drain, then refrigerate to cool.

2 Meanwhile, cook the gingered vegetables. Put all the vegetables into a steamer with the ginger, cover and cook over boiling water for 7 minutes or until tender.

3 Remove the central choke of each artichoke and fill with the vegetables.

4 To make the sauce, place all the ingredients in a food processor or blender and purée until smooth. To serve, pour some sauce over each artichoke.

# Courgette cakes with minted sauce and salsa

alcohol free ✓ | citrus free ✗ | dairy free ✗ | gluten free ✗ | wheat free ✗

**Serves 4**
**Preparation time: 20 minutes, plus chilling**
**Cooking time: 6–8 minutes**

**Per serving**
Energy 435 kcals/1822 kJ | Protein 12 g | Carbohydrate 48 g | Fat 23 g
Fibre 4 g

500 g (1 lb) courgettes, finely grated
2 tablespoons mayonnaise
300 g (10 oz) fresh breadcrumbs
½ teaspoon ground cumin
½ teaspoon ground coriander
¼ teaspoon cayenne pepper
vegetable oil, for shallow-frying

Minted Sauce:
4 tablespoons finely chopped mint
finely grated rind and juice of 1 lime
150 ml (¼ pint) Greek yogurt

Salsa:
2 ripe plum tomatoes or vine tomatoes, deseeded and finely diced
½ cucumber, deseeded and finely diced
1 small red onion, finely chopped
1 teaspoon white wine vinegar
1 teaspoon sugar
salt and pepper

1 Put the grated courgettes into a colander and squeeze out as much liquid from them as possible. Transfer them to a bowl. Add the mayonnaise, breadcrumbs, cumin, coriander and cayenne pepper. Season with salt and pepper to taste and mix well. Set aside.

2 Mix the ingredients for the minted yogurt sauce in a serving bowl with salt and pepper to taste. Cover and chill until ready to serve.

3 Combine the ingredients for the salsa in a serving bowl. Cover and chill until ready to serve.

4 Divide the courgette mixture into 12 portions. Heat the oil in a large nonstick frying pan. Put as many portions as will fit in the pan, flattening each one to form a thick cake. Fry the cakes for 3–4 minutes on each side or until lightly browned. Drain on kitchen paper and keep hot until all the mixture is cooked.

5 Serve the courgette cakes hot with the chilled sauce and salsa.

# Salads, vegetables and side dishes

## Insalata mista

alcohol free ✓ I citrus free ✗ I dairy free ✓ I gluten free ✓ I wheat free ✓

**Serves 4**
**Preparation time: 10 minutes**

**Per serving**
Energy 310 kcals/1274 kJ I Protein 2 g I Carbohydrate 2 g I Fat 33 g
Fibre 1 g

salad leaves, such as lettuce, endive and radicchio
basil or rocket leaves

Dressing:
juice of 1 lemon
4 tablespoons white or red wine vinegar
175 ml (6 fl oz) Italian olive oil
salt and pepper

**1** First make the dressing. Combine the lemon juice, vinegar and salt in a jug. Stir to dissolve the salt, then whisk in the olive oil. Leave to stand for 5 minutes, then season with pepper. Taste and add more salt if required.

**2** Tear the salad leaves into pieces and arrange them in a salad bowl. Shred the basil or rocket and mix with the salad leaves. Toss with the dressing and serve immediately.

# Pasta and avocado salad with tomato dressing

alcohol free ✓ | citrus free ✓ | dairy free ✓ | gluten free ✗ | wheat free ✗

**Serves 4**
**Preparation time: 15 minutes, plus standing time**
**Cooking time: 10–12 minutes**

**Per serving**
Energy 392 kcals/1636 kJ | Protein 7 g | Carbohydrate 35 g | Fat 26 g
Fibre 3 g

175 g (6 oz) small pasta shells
1 quantity Tomato, Garlic and Summer Herb Dressing (see
  page 136)
2 ripe avocados
salt and pepper

**1** Bring a large saucepan of salted water to the boil, add the small
pasta shells and cook according to the packet instructions. Drain
in a colander and cool under cold running water. Drain well and
transfer to a bowl.

**2** Add the dressing to the pasta and toss well, to coat the pasta
completely. Season to taste with salt and pepper.

**3** To serve, halve and stone the avocados, then peel and slice them
lengthways. Divide the pasta salad between 4 serving plates and
arrange the avocado slices on top.

# Tomato, garlic and summer herb dressing

alcohol free ✓ | citrus free ✓ | dairy free ✓ | gluten free ✓ | wheat free ✓

**Makes 350 ml/12 fl oz**
**Preparation time: 15 minutes, plus standing time**

**Per serving**
Energy 418 kcals/1720 kJ | Protein 2 g | Carbohydrate 3 g | Fat 44 g
Fibre 1 g

500 g/1 lb ripe tomatoes, skinned, seeded and finely diced
2 garlic cloves, finely chopped
2 tablespoons balsamic vinegar
4 tablespoons extra-virgin olive oil
6 large basil leaves, finely shredded
3 tablespoons chopped mixed herbs (e.g. dill, chervil, chives, parsley, mint)
salt and pepper

**1** Place the tomatoes in a bowl with the garlic, balsamic vinegar and olive oil. Stir well.

**2** Add the shredded basil to the tomato mixture with the mixed herbs. Stir in salt and pepper to taste. Mix thoroughly. Leave to stand for at least 30 minutes before using, to allow the flavours to develop and mingle.

# Warm salad of red peppers and scallops

alcohol free ✓ | citrus free ✗ | dairy free ✓ | gluten free ✓ | wheat free ✓

**Serves 4**
**Preparation time: 10–15 minutes**
**Cooking time: about 10 minutes**

**Per serving**
Energy 213 kcals/892 kJ | Protein 22 g | Carbohydrate 6 g | Fat 11 g
Fibre 1 g

2 tablespoons lemon juice
3 tablespoons olive oil, more if needed
2 red peppers, cored, deseeded and cut into thin strips
mixed salad leaves
375 g (12 oz) scallops, cleaned
50 g (2 oz) black olives, pitted and quartered
2 tablespoons snipped chives
salt and pepper

**1** In a small bowl, combine the lemon juice, 2 tablespoons of the oil and salt and pepper. Set aside.

**2** Heat the remaining oil in a frying pan over a moderate heat. Add the red peppers with a pinch of salt and sauté for 5 minutes until tender. Set aside. Arrange the salad on individual plates.

**3** Rinse the scallops and pat dry with kitchen paper. Season them with salt and pepper and arrange in one layer in the top of a steamer set over boiling water. Cover and steam over a high heat for about 3 minutes until tender. Drain on kitchen paper.

**4** To serve, arrange the warm scallops on the salad leaves. Arrange the red peppers, olives and chives around the scallops. Whisk the dressing and spoon over the salad. Serve immediately.

# Potato gnocchi

alcohol free ✓ I citrus free ✓ I dairy free ✗ I gluten free ✗ I wheat free ✗

**Serves 4**
**Preparation time: 30 minutes**
**Cooking time: 35 minutes**

**Per serving**
Energy 524 kcals/2212 kJ I Protein 13 g I Carbohydrate 95 g I Fat 13 g
Fibre 6 g

1 kg (2 lb) floury potatoes, such as Desirée, unpeeled
50 g (2 oz) butter
1 egg, beaten
250–300 g (8–10 oz) plain white flour
semolina flour or plain white flour, for sprinkling
salt

To Serve:
melted butter
chopped sage
freshly grated Parmesan cheese

1 Cook the potatoes in boiling water for 20–30 minutes until very tender. Drain well. Alternatively, bake them in the oven until tender. Holding the potatoes in a tea towel, peel off the skins, then pass the potatoes through a potato ricer or sieve into a bowl.

2 Add 1 teaspoon salt, the butter, beaten egg and half the flour. Lightly mix together, then turn out on to a floured board. Gradually knead the rest of the flour into the dough until it is smooth, soft and a little sticky.

3 Roll the dough into long sausages, about 2.5 cm (1 inch) thick, and cut them into 1.5 cm (¾ inch) pieces. Take each piece and roll it over the back of a fork with your floured thumb so the gnocchi form ridges on one side and an indentation on the other. Spread out the gnocchi on a tea towel sprinkled with semolina or plain flour.

4 Cook the gnocchi in a large pan of boiling salted water for 2–3 minutes or until they float to the surface. Remove with a slotted spoon and toss with melted butter, chopped sage and plenty of grated Parmesan.

# Gingered rice
# with carrots and tomatoes

alcohol free ✓  |  citrus free ✗  |  dairy free ✓  |  gluten free ✓  |  wheat free ✓

**Serves 4**
**Preparation time: 15 minutes**
**Cooking time: 25 minutes**

**Per serving**
Energy 440 kcals/1840 kJ  |  Protein 8 g  |  Carbohydrate 60 g  |  Fat 19 g
Fibre 5 g

250 g (8 oz) basmati rice
4 tablespoons extra-virgin olive oil
2 garlic cloves, crushed
1 tablespoon grated fresh root ginger
4 carrots, sliced thinly
4 ripe tomatoes, skinned, deseeded and diced
2 cinnamon sticks, bruised
seeds from 3 cardamom pods, bruised
1 dried red chilli
1 tablespoon lemon juice
50 g (2 oz) flaked almonds, toasted
salt and pepper

**1** Cook the rice in plenty of boiling salted water for 5 minutes.
Drain, refresh under cold water and drain again. Spread out on a
large baking sheet and set aside to dry.

**2** Heat the oil in a wok or large frying pan, add the garlic, ginger
and carrots and fry for 10 minutes. Add the tomatoes and spices
and cook for a further 5 minutes.

**3** Stir in the rice, lemon juice, almonds and salt and pepper to
taste, and stir-fry for 3–4 minutes. Serve at once.

# Main meals

## Chicken and pasta twist bake

alcohol free ✓ | citrus free ✓ | dairy free ✕ | gluten free ✕ | wheat free ✕

**Serves 4**
**Preparation time: about 15 minutes**
**Cooking time: about 20 minutes**

**Per serving**
Energy 354 kcals/1500 kJ | Protein 27 g | Carbohydrate 58 g | Fat 4 g
Fibre 4 g

40 g (1½ oz) plain flour, sieved
600 ml (1 pint) skimmed milk
200 g (7 oz) tricoloured pasta twists
250 g (8 oz) boneless, skinless chicken breast, cooked and diced
50 g (2 oz) fresh wholemeal breadcrumbs
salt and pepper

**1** Blend the flour with the milk in a saucepan and bring to the boil over a gentle heat, stirring constantly until the sauce thickens. Simmer for 1 minute, stirring frequently, then season generously with pepper.

**2** Meanwhile, cook the pasta twists in a large pan of salted boiling water according to packet instructions until tender. Drain well.

**3** Stir the chicken into the sauce, then pour into a 2.5 litre (4 pint) shallow ovenproof dish. Spoon the pasta twists over the sauce, pressing them in lightly, without submerging them completely. Sprinkle the breadcrumbs over the pasta and bake in a preheated oven, 190°C (375°F), Gas Mark 5, for about 20 minutes, until the breadcrumbs are golden and crisp.

# Chicken risotto

alcohol free ✓ | citrus free ✓ | dairy free ✕ | gluten free ✓ | wheat free ✓

**Serves 4**
**Preparation time: 10 minutes**
**Cooking time: 30–35 minutes**

**Per serving**
Energy 507 kcals/2135 kJ | Protein 22 g | Carbohydrate 66 g | Fat 19 g
Fibre 2 g

40 g (1½ oz) butter
2 tablespoons olive oil
2 boneless, skinless chicken breasts, diced
½ onion, very finely chopped
1 garlic clove, finely chopped
1–2 fresh red chillies, deseeded and very finely chopped (optional)
300 g (10 oz) arborio risotto rice
1 litre (1¾ pints) boiling Chicken Stock (see page 175), kept
    simmering
3 tablespoons freshly grated Parmesan cheese
salt and pepper

**1** Melt 15 g (½ oz) of the butter with the oil in a saucepan, add the
diced chicken and fry gently for 2–3 minutes. Add the onion and
fry for 5 minutes until soft but not coloured. Add the garlic and
chilli, if using, and fry until the garlic is golden.

**2** Add the rice to the pan and stir for 1–2 minutes. Add the hot
stock, a ladleful at a time, stirring constantly and allowing the
liquid to be absorbed before adding more. This will take about
25 minutes, leaving the rice creamy but still firm to the bite.

**3** Add the Parmesan to the rice. Season with salt and pepper, and
stir in the remaining butter.

# Tomato and mushroom risotto

alcohol free ✓  |  citrus free ✓  |  dairy free ✗  |  gluten free ✓  |  wheat free ✓

**Serves 4**
**Preparation time: 10 minutes**
**Cooking time: 30 minutes**

**Per serving**
Energy 577 kcals/2430 kJ  |  Protein 13 g  |  Carbohydrate 92 g  |  Fat 20 g
Fibre 5 g

75 g (3 oz) unsalted butter
1 onion, finely chopped
250 g (8 oz) chestnut mushrooms, sliced
3 large tomatoes, skinned and chopped
400 g (13 oz) arborio rice
1 litre (1¾ pints) Chicken Stock (see page 179), kept simmering
40 g (1½ oz) freshly grated Parmesan cheese
salt and pepper
thyme sprigs, to garnish

**1** Melt three-quarters of the butter in a large heavy-based
saucepan. Add the onion and cook over a low heat, stirring, for 5
minutes. Add the mushrooms and three-quarters of the tomatoes
and continue to stir over low heat for a further 5 minutes.

**2** Add the rice and stir to coat with the butter. Increase the heat
and brown the rice, stirring constantly, for 30 seconds. Pour in a
ladleful of the hot stock, reduce the heat to medium-low and stir
until absorbed. Continue adding stock, a ladleful at a time,
stirring constantly and allowing it to be absorbed, until the rice is
creamy but firm to the bite. Stir in the remaining butter and the
Parmesan and cook until the cheese has melted. Season to taste,
transfer to warmed bowls and serve immediately, sprinkled with
the remaining tomatoes and thyme sprigs.

# Saffron millet and lentils with radicchio

alcohol free ✓ I citrus free ✓ I dairy free ✗ I gluten free ✓ I wheat free ✓

**Serves 4–6**
**Preparation time: 10 minutes**
**Cooking time: 50 minutes**

**Per serving**
Energy 336 kcals/1408 kJ I Protein 10 g I Carbohydrate 48 g I Fat 12 g
Fibre 2 g

pinch of saffron threads
900 ml (1½ pints) boiling vegetable stock
125 g (4 oz) Puy lentils, rinsed
125 g (4 oz) millet
50 g (2 oz) butter
1 leek, sliced
2 garlic cloves, sliced
1 teaspoon ground cinnamon
50 g (2 oz) currants
1 small head radicchio, shredded
salt and pepper

**1** Soak the saffron threads in the boiling vegetable stock for 10 minutes.

**2** Meanwhile, put the lentils into a saucepan and add enough water to cover the lentils by about 2.5 cm (1 inch). Bring to the boil, and boil the lentils rapidly for 10 minutes, then drain.

**3** Place the millet in a small frying pan and heat gently until the grains start to turn golden.

**4** Melt the butter in a saucepan, add the leek, garlic and cinnamon and fry for 3 minutes. Stir in the lentils and millet and then pour in the saffron stock. Bring to the boil, cover and simmer gently for 30 minutes until the lentils and millet are tender.

**5** Stir in the currants and shredded radicchio and heat through for 5 minutes. Season to taste with salt and pepper and serve at once.

# Thai noodles with vegetables and tofu

alcohol free ✓ I citrus free ✗ I dairy free ✓ I gluten free ✗ I wheat free ✗

**Serves 4**
**Preparation time: 20 minutes, plus marinating**
**Cooking time: 40 minutes**

**Per serving**
Energy 296 kcals/1246 kJ I Protein 18 g I Carbohydrate 40 g I Fat 9 g
Fibre 4 g

250 g (8 oz) tofu, cubed
2 tablespoons dark soy sauce
1 teaspoon grated lime rind
1.75 litres (3 pints) vegetable stock
2 slices fresh root ginger
2 garlic cloves
2 coriander sprigs
2 lemon grass stalks, crushed
1 red chilli, bruised
175 g (6 oz) dried egg noodles
125 g (4 oz) shiitake or button mushrooms, sliced
2 large carrots, cut into matchsticks
125 g (4 oz) sugar snap peas
125 g (4 oz) Chinese cabbage, shredded
2 tablespoons chopped coriander
salt and pepper

**1** Put the tofu in a shallow dish with the soy sauce and lime rind, and leave to marinate for 30 minutes.

**2** Meanwhile, put the vegetable stock into a large saucepan and add the ginger, garlic, coriander sprigs, lemon grass and chilli. Bring the mixture to the boil, then reduce the heat, cover the pan and simmer gently for 30 minutes.

**3** Strain the cooked vegetable stock into another saucepan, return it to the heat and plunge in the noodles. Add the sliced mushrooms and marinaded tofu with any remaining marinade. Reduce the heat and simmer gently for 4 minutes.

**4** Stir in the carrots, sugar snap peas, shredded Chinese cabbage and chopped coriander and cook for a further 3–4 minutes, until all the vegetables are just tender. Taste and adjust the seasoning, if necessary. Serve at once.

# Tagliatelle with tomato sauce

alcohol free ✕ | citrus free ✓ | dairy free ✕ | gluten free ✕ | wheat free ✕

**Serves 6**
**Preparation time: 10 minutes**
**Cooking time: 20 minutes**

**Per serving**
Energy 256 kcals/1080 kJ | Protein 8 g | Carbohydrate 39 g | Fat 7 g
Fibre 4 g

2 tablespoons olive oil
2 onions, chopped
2 garlic cloves, crushed
500 g (1 lb) tomatoes, skinned and chopped
2 tablespoons tomato purée
1 teaspoon sugar
125 ml (4 fl oz) dry white wine
a few ripe olives, pitted and quartered
a handful of torn basil leaves
250 g (8 oz) dried tagliatelle
25 g (1 oz) freshly grated Parmesan cheese (optional)
salt and pepper

**1** Heat half the oil in a large frying pan. Add the onions and garlic and sauté gently over a low heat until tender and slightly coloured, stirring occasionally.

**2** Add the tomatoes and tomato purée with the sugar and wine, stirring well. Cook over a gentle heat until the mixture is thick and reduced. Stir in the olives and basil and season to taste with salt and plenty of pepper.

**3** Meanwhile, add the tagliatelle to a large pan of boiling salted water. Boil rapidly until just tender.

**4** Drain the tagliatelle immediately, mixing in the remaining oil and a generous grinding of pepper. Arrange the pasta on 4 warmed plates and top with the tomato sauce, mixing it into the tagliatelle. Serve sprinkled with Parmesan cheese, if liked.

# Lamb kebabs

alcohol free ✓ | citrus free ✗ | dairy free ✓ | gluten free ✓ | wheat free ✓

**Serves 6**
**Preparation time: 30 minutes, plus marinating**
**Cooking time: 10–15 minutes**

**Per serving**
Energy 430 kcals/1784 kJ | Protein 30 g | Carbohydrate 1 g | Fat 34 g
Fibre 0 g

1 kg (2 lb) boned shoulder of lamb, cut into 5 cm (2 inch) cubes
lemon wedges, to serve

Marinade:
3 tablespoons olive oil
2 tablespoons lemon juice
1 garlic clove, crushed
1½ tablespoons paprika
1 teaspoon ground cumin
1 teaspoon ground coriander
1 teaspoon tomato purée

**1** Put the lamb into a bowl. Mix together all the marinade ingredients, add to the lamb and stir to mix thoroughly. Cover and leave at room temperature for 2 hours, or overnight in the refrigerator. If you put the lamb in the refrigerator, return it to room temperature 1 hour before cooking.

**2** Remove the lamb from the marinade, pat dry and thread on to 6 long skewers. Cook under a preheated grill for 10–15 minutes, turning occasionally and brushing with any remaining marinade, until browned on the outside but still pink inside.

**3** Serve on a bed of salad, if you like, with lemon wedges.

# Sea bass with fennel

alcohol free ✓ | citrus free ✓ | dairy free ✓ | gluten free ✓ | wheat free ✓

**Serves 4**
**Preparation time: 5 minutes**
**Cooking time: 45–50 minutes**

**Per serving**
Energy 362 kcals/1508 kJ | Protein 39 g | Carbohydrate 2 g | Fat 22 g
Fibre 0 g

2 large fennel bulbs
6 tablespoons olive oil
8 tablespoons water
2 sea bass, about 500 g (1 lb) each, filleted
salt and pepper
carrot matchsticks, to garnish

**1** Cut the fennel bulbs lengthways into 1 cm (½ inch) slices. Pour the oil into a wok, add the fennel and water and bring to the boil. Cover and simmer for 30 minutes, until the fennel is very tender, stirring occasionally.

**2** Remove the lid, season the fennel with salt and pepper and boil until all the water has evaporated and the fennel is golden brown. Transfer to a warmed plate and keep hot.

**3** Season the fish with salt and pepper, add to the wok and baste with the hot oil. Cover and cook for 7–8 minutes. Turn the fish over, baste again and cook for a further 5–6 minutes.

**4** Arrange the fennel on a warmed serving dish. Place the fish on the fennel and pour the cooking juices around and over the fish and serve immediately, garnished with carrot matchsticks.

# Halibut on a bed of vegetables

alcohol free ✓  |  citrus free ✓  |  dairy free ✕  |  gluten free ✓  |  wheat free ✓

**Serves 2**
**Preparation time: 15 minutes**
**Cooking time: 25 minutes**

**Per serving**
Energy 496 kcals/2067 kJ  |  Protein 36 g  |  Carbohydrate 10 g  |  Fat 35 g
Fibre 5 g

2 tablespoons olive oil
½ red pepper, cored, deseeded and roughly chopped
½ green pepper, cored, deseeded and roughly chopped
50 g (2 oz) mushrooms, sliced
1 courgette, sliced lengthways into 3 cm (1½ inch) pieces
½ aubergine, sliced lengthways and cut into 3 cm (1½ inch) pieces
2 tomatoes, skinned and chopped
1 tablespoon tomato purée
2 halibut steaks, about 150–175 g (5–6 oz) each
50 g (2 oz) butter
2 tablespoons chopped mixed parsley, tarragon and chives
salt and pepper

**1** Heat the oil in a large saucepan, add the red and green peppers, mushrooms, courgette, aubergine, tomatoes and tomato purée and fry for 15–20 minutes over a moderate heat, stirring occasionally.

**2** Meanwhile, line a baking sheet with a large piece of foil, allowing sufficient to fold over the fish comfortably. Place the fish on the foil, dot with butter, sprinkle with the herbs and season with salt and pepper. Fold the foil loosely over the fish and bake in a preheated oven, 200°C (400°F), Gas Mark 6, for 18–20 minutes until cooked through.

**3** When the fish and vegetables are cooked, season to taste with salt and pepper and add more herbs or tomato purée if necessary. Spoon the vegetables on to warmed plates and put the halibut on top. Serve immediately.

# Fresh tuna with tomatoes

alcohol free ✓  |  citrus free ✓  |  dairy free ✓  |  gluten free ✕  |  wheat free ✕

**Serves 4**
**Preparation time: 15 minutes**
**Cooking time: 30 minutes**

**Per serving**
Energy 339 kcals/1419 kJ  |  Protein 38 g  |  Carbohydrate 7 g  |  Fat 18 g
Fibre 3 g

4 tuna steaks, about 150 g (5 oz) each
flour, for dusting
3 tablespoons olive oil
1 onion, chopped
2 garlic cloves, crushed
750 g (1½ lb) tomatoes, skinned and chopped
2 tablespoons chopped parsley
a few basil leaves, shredded
1 bay leaf
4 anchovy fillets, mashed
8 black olives
salt and pepper

1 Wash the tuna steaks and pat dry with kitchen paper. Season with salt and plenty of pepper, then dust the steaks lightly with flour.

2 Heat half the olive oil in a large shallow frying pan and sauté the tuna steaks until golden on one side. Flip them over and cook the other side until golden. Carefully remove them from the pan and transfer to a dish and keep warm.

3 Heat the remaining oil in the pan, add the onion and garlic and sauté for about 3 minutes, until soft and golden. Add the tomatoes, parsley, basil, bay leaf and mashed anchovies and stir well. Heat through gently, allowing the tomatoes to keep their shape.

4 Return the tuna to the pan, season to taste with salt and pepper and simmer gently for 15 minutes, turning once. Turn off the heat. Add the olives and leave to stand for 5 minutes.

5 To serve, discard the bay leaf, arrange the vegetables on warmed plates and place the tuna steaks on top.

# Smoked haddock and basmati rice salad

alcohol free ✓ | citrus free ✕ | dairy free ✕ | gluten free ✓ | wheat free ✓

**Serves 4**
**Preparation time: 15 minutes, plus cooling**
**Cooking time: 20 minutes**

**Per serving**
Energy 490 kcals/2054 kJ | Protein 35 g | Carbohydrate 42 g | Fat 21 g
Fibre 1 g

175 g (6 oz) basmati rice, cooked
3 hard-boiled eggs, chopped
2 tablespoons chopped coriander or parsley
1 red or yellow pepper
500 g (1 lb) smoked haddock fillet
1 onion, chopped
1 bay leaf
1 tablespoon lightly crushed coriander seeds
1 teaspoon lightly crushed cumin seeds
300 ml (½ pint) milk

Dressing:
1 garlic clove, crushed (optional)
3 tablespoons mayonnaise
pepper

To Garnish:
lemon wedges
coriander sprigs

1 Put the cooked basmati rice, chopped eggs and the coriander or parsley into a large salad bowl and set aside.

2 Halve the pepper and remove the seeds. Cook under a hot grill, skin side up, until the skin is blackened and blistered. Cool slightly, then remove the charred skin. Cut the flesh into thin strips and set aside.

3 Meanwhile, put the smoked haddock, onion, bay leaf, coriander seeds and cumin seeds into a large frying pan, pour in the milk and bring to the boil. Immediately lower the heat, until the liquid is barely simmering, and cook for about 8–10 minutes until the fish flakes easily and is cooked through. Using a slotted spoon, transfer the fish to a plate and allow to cool. Remove the skin and any obvious bones and flake the fish into bite-sized pieces. Add to the rice mixture.

4 To make the dressing, strain the fish cooking liquid and return to the pan. Add the crushed garlic, if using. Cook over a high heat for 1–2 minutes or until reduced by half. Remove from the heat and add the mayonnaise, blending well until smooth. Season with freshly ground black pepper (you shouldn't need salt as the fish is quite salty), set aside and allow to cool.

5 To serve, add the dressing to the salad and toss lightly to mix. Scatter the reserved pepper strips over the top. Serve the salad garnished with lemon wedges and coriander sprigs.

# Desserts

## Mango and passion fruit sorbet

alcohol free ✓ | citrus free ✗ | dairy free ✓ | gluten free ✓ | wheat free ✓

**Serves 4**
**Preparation time: 10–15 minutes, plus cooling and freezing**
**Cooking time: about 4 minutes**

**Per serving**
Energy 125 kcals/535 kJ | Protein 2 g | Carbohydrate 31 g | Fat 0 g
Fibre 2 g

2 ripe mangoes
4 passion fruit
1 tablespoon lemon juice
75 g (3 oz) caster sugar
150 ml (¼ pint) water
1–2 egg whites (optional)

1 Cut the skin from the mangoes and cut the pulp from the stones. Halve the passion fruit and scoop out all the pulp. Put the pulp into a food processor or blender and work to a purée or rub through a sieve.

2 Put the lemon juice, sugar and water into a saucepan and heat just until the sugar has dissolved. Stir into the fruit purée and allow to cool.

3 Turn the mixture into a freezer container, cover and freeze until firm, stirring once or twice during freezing.

4 If liked, whisk 1–2 egg whites until stiff, then fold them into the fruit purée when it is slightly frozen. This extends the purée and gives a greater volume, but the egg whites do take away some of the natural fruit flavour.

5 Transfer the sorbet to the refrigerator 15 minutes before serving to soften.

# Mighty muesli

alcohol free ✓ I citrus free ✓ I dairy free ✕ I gluten free ✕ I wheat free ✓

**Serves 6**
**Preparation time: 5 minutes, plus cooling**
**Cooking time: 20 minutes**

**Per serving**
Energy 298 kcals/1250 kJ I Protein 9 g I Carbohydrate 36 g I Fat 14 g
Fibre 3 g

50 g (2 oz) sunflower seeds
50 g (2 oz) pumpkin seeds
1 tablespoon sesame seeds
1 tablespoon desiccated coconut
2 tablespoons linseeds
75 g (3 oz) sultanas
175 g (6 oz) rolled oats
2 tablespoons soft light brown sugar or 1 tablespoon clear honey or
   maple syrup

To Serve:
assorted peeled and sliced fruit, such as papayas, mangoes, bananas,
   peaches, strawberries and apples
thick yogurt

1 Mix together the sunflower, pumpkin and sesame seeds on a baking sheet with the desiccated coconut and roast in a preheated oven, 200°C (400°F), Gas Mark 6, for 5–8 minutes or until beginning to brown. Remove from the oven and put into a bowl with the linseeds and sultanas.

2 Mix the rolled oats with the sugar, honey or maple syrup and spread on a baking sheet. Cook the oats in the oven for 10–15 minutes or until they begin to brown and stick together in clumps, stirring occasionally.

3 Remove the oats from the oven and leave to cool for 5 minutes, then stir them to separate the clumps. Leave the oats to cool completely, then stir them into the seeds and sultanas. When completely cold, transfer the muesli to an airtight container.

4 Serve the muesli over thickly sliced mango, papaya and banana, and add a large spoonful of yogurt.

# Stuffed figs

alcohol free ✓  |  citrus free ✓  |  dairy free ✓  |  gluten free ✓  |  wheat free ✓

**Serves 4**
**Preparation time: 10–15 minutes**

**Per serving**
Energy 120 kcals/518 kJ  |  Protein 4 g  |  Carbohydrate 202 g  |  Fat 3 g
Fibre 5 g

12 ripe fresh figs, preferably purple ones
3 tablespoons ground almonds
125 g (4 oz) fresh raspberries
1 tablespoon clear honey
4 vine leaves, soaked in warm water and dried, to serve

**1** Snip off any excess stalk from each fig. Make a criss-cross cut down from the stalk end and carefully ease the cut open.

**2** In a bowl, mix the ground almonds together with the raspberries and honey.

**3** Place a vine leaf, spread out flat, on each serving plate. Arrange 3 figs on top of each one and fill with the raspberry and almond purée.

# 7 Self-help nutrition

It is vital for everyone to eat a well-balanced diet. However, people with IBS need to pay special attention because diet can play a significant part in triggering or alleviating symptoms.

IBS sufferers often find symptoms are best controlled by consuming several smaller meals a day rather than three heavy meals. This chapter contains ideas for starters and salads, light meals, main meals and desserts, all designed to boost your overall health and wellbeing.

Because everyone's symptoms are different there may be some recipes that you find suit you better than others. Don't feel bound by the ingredients: if a recipe contains something that disagrees with you, feel free to adapt it. The emphasis is on restoring an enjoyment of food through the creation of healthy delicious dishes that look as good as they taste.

# Soups and starters

## Green lentils with egg and spiced mayonnaise

alcohol free ✓ | citrus free ✗ | dairy free ✓ | gluten free ✓ | wheat free ✓

**Serves 4**
**Preparation time: 10 minutes**

**Per serving**
Energy 558 kcals/2310 kJ | Protein 16 g | Carbohydrate 48 g | Fat 18 g
Fibre 2 g

425 g (14 oz) can green lentils
4 spring onions, finely chopped
2 tablespoons chopped coriander
1 tablespoon olive oil
1 teaspoon lemon or lime juice
4 hard-boiled eggs
salt and pepper
fine strips of red chilli, to garnish (optional)

Dressing (optional):
6 tablespoons mayonnaise
1–2 tablespoons mild curry paste

**1** Rinse the lentils and drain thoroughly. Place in a bowl with the spring onions, coriander, olive oil and lemon or lime juice. Season with salt and pepper and mix well.

**2** To make the dressing, if using, stir together the mayonnaise and mild curry paste until smooth.

**3** To serve the salad, arrange piles of the lentil mixture on 4 individual plates. Top each one with a dollop of dressing and an egg, halved or sliced. Garnish each serving with a few strips of red chilli, if using.

# Vietnamese salad rolls with dipping sauce

alcohol free ✓ | citrus free ✕ | dairy free ✓ | gluten free ✓ | wheat free ✓

**Serves 4**
**Preparation time: 15 minutes**

**Per serving**
Energy 133 kcals/555 kJ | Protein 3 g | Carbohydrate 28 g | Fat 0 g
Fibre 3 g

12 small rice paper spring roll wrappers
1 carrot, cut into thin matchsticks
1 cucumber, halved lengthways, deseeded and cut into thin
  matchsticks
125 g (4 oz) bean sprouts
2 spring onions, finely shredded
15 g (½ oz) mint leaves
15 g (½ oz) coriander leaves

Dipping Sauce:
2 tablespoons Thai fish sauce
3 tablespoons lime juice
2 teaspoons caster sugar
1 small red chilli, deseeded and finely sliced (optional)

1 Soak the spring roll wrappers in hot water for 1–2 minutes or until softened. Drain well.

2 Lay the wrappers on a clean work surface or board and cover with a damp tea towel.

3 Divide the carrot, cucumber, bean sprouts, spring onions, mint and coriander evenly between the wrappers. Fold and roll the wrappers around the salad filling to enclose it in neat packages. Place on a board and cover with a damp tea towel until ready to serve.

4 Mix together all the ingredients for the dipping sauce and pour into a small bowl. Arrange the salad rolls on a large platter or individual plates and serve with the dipping sauce.

# Fava

alcohol free ✓ | citrus free ✕ | dairy free ✓ | gluten free ✓ | wheat free ✓

**Serves 4**
**Preparation time: 5 minutes**
**Cooking time: 40–45 minutes**

**Per serving**
Energy 170 kcals/709 kJ | Protein 3 g | Carbohydrate 8 g | Fat 14 g
Fibre 2 g

50 g (2 oz) yellow split peas, rinsed
4 tablespoons extra-virgin olive oil
1 small garlic clove, crushed
1 tablespoon lemon juice
¼ teaspoon ground cumin
½ teaspoon mustard powder
pinch of cayenne pepper
salt and pepper

To Garnish:
1 tablespoon chopped parsley
1 tablespoon chopped red pepper
pinch of cayenne pepper
1 tablespoon extra-virgin olive oil

1 Put the split peas into a saucepan and add enough cold water to cover them by about 2.5 cm (1 inch). Bring to the boil and simmer over a low heat, stirring frequently, for 30–35 minutes, until all the water is absorbed and the split peas are cooked. Leave to cool slightly.

2 Place the split peas in a food processor or blender with all the remaining ingredients, season to taste with salt and pepper and process until smooth, adding 2–3 tablespoons of boiling water if the mixture is too thick.

3 Transfer to a serving dish and sprinkle with the parsley, red pepper and cayenne. Drizzle with the olive oil. Serve with a selection of prepared raw vegetables and warm pitta bread for dipping.

# Yellow pepper soup

alcohol free ✓ I citrus free ✓ I dairy free ✗ I gluten free ✓ I wheat free ✓

**Serves 8**
**Preparation time: 15–20 minutes**
**Cooking time: 50–55 minutes**

**Per serving**
Energy 88 kcals/367 kJ I Protein 1 g I Carbohydrate 9 g I Fat 5 g
Fibre 2 g

3 yellow peppers, cored and deseeded
50 g (2 oz) butter or margarine
1 small onion, chopped
1.2 litres (2 pints) vegetable stock
1 teaspoon mild curry powder
¼ teaspoon turmeric
1 tablespoon chopped coriander
300 g (10 oz) potatoes, chopped
salt

1 Chop one pepper finely and place it in a small saucepan, then roughly chop the remaining two peppers.

2 Melt 25 g (1 oz) of the butter or margarine in another saucepan and cook the onion and roughly chopped peppers for 5 minutes, stirring frequently. Stir in the stock, curry powder, turmeric and coriander, then add the potatoes. Season with salt. Bring to the boil, then lower the heat and simmer, partially covered, for 40–45 minutes, or until the vegetables are very soft.

3 Melt the remaining butter with the finely chopped pepper in the small pan. Cook over a gentle heat until the pepper is very soft. Reserve for the garnish.

4 Purée the onion, pepper and potato mixture in batches in a food processor or blender until very smooth. Return the purée to a clean saucepan and reheat gently. Serve the soup in warmed soup plates or bowls, garnished with a little of the sautéed chopped pepper.

# Avgolemono

alcohol free ✓  |  citrus free ✕  |  dairy free ✓  |  gluten free ✓  |  wheat free ✓

**Serves 6**
**Preparation time: about 10 minutes**
**Cooking time: 25 minutes**

**Per serving**
Energy 55 kcals/234 kJ  |  Protein 3 g  |  Carbohydrate 7 g  |  Fat 2 g
Fibre 0 g

1.5 litres (2½ pints) Chicken Stock (see page 175)
50 g (2 oz) white long-grain rice
2 eggs
2–3 tablespoons lemon juice
1 tablespoon chopped parsley (optional)
salt and pepper

**1** Combine the stock and the rice in a saucepan with ½ teaspoon of salt and bring to the boil. Stir, lower the heat, cover the pan and simmer for 20 minutes. Stir once more.

**2** Beat the eggs in a small bowl, then whisk in the lemon juice. Add a ladleful of stock, beat, and then add another ladleful of stock and beat once more.

**3** Bring the remaining stock and rice mixture to the boil. Briefly remove the saucepan from the heat and add the egg and lemon mixture. Stir well, lower the heat and simmer for 2 minutes, adding salt and pepper to taste. Sprinkle with the parsley, if using. Serve at once in warmed bowls.

# Fennel soup

alcohol free ✓ I citrus free ✓ I dairy free ✗ I gluten free ✗ I wheat free ✗

**Serves 4**
**Preparation time: 5 minutes**
**Cooking time: 25 minutes**

**Per serving**
Energy 38 kcals/158 kJ I Protein 3 g I Carbohydrate 4 g I Fat 1 g
Fibre 1 g

2 fennel bulbs, with leaves
1 onion, finely chopped
600 ml (1 pint) Chicken Stock (see page 179)
150 ml (¼ pint) skimmed milk
1 teaspoon pesto
salt and pepper
small wholemeal croûtons, to serve

**1** Remove the feathery leaves from the fennel, and reserve for a
garnish. Cut the bulbs into shreds.

**2** Put the fennel into a saucepan with the onion, chicken stock,
skimmed milk and salt and pepper to taste. Bring to the boil then
lower the heat and simmer gently for about 20 minutes, until the
fennel is just tender.

**3** Allow the soup to cool slightly, then purée in a food processor or
blender until smooth. Return to a clean saucepan, add the pesto
and heat through gently.

**4** Ladle the soup into warmed bowls. Garnish with the fennel
leaves, and serve with wholemeal croûtons.

# Tomato, orange and tarragon soup

alcohol free ✓ I citrus free ✗ I dairy free ✓ I gluten free ✓ I wheat free ✓

**Serves 8**
**Preparation time: 15 minutes**
**Cooking time: about 30 minutes**

**Per serving**
Energy 84 kcals/358 kJ I Protein 2 g I Carbohydrate 15 g I Fat 2 g
Fibre 4 g

1 tablespoon vegetable oil
1 onion, sliced
175 g (6 oz) potatoes, diced
1.75 kg (3½ lb) tomatoes, chopped
2 tablespoons chopped tarragon
1 garlic clove, crushed
500 ml (17 fl oz) Chicken Stock (see opposite)
250 ml (8 fl oz) orange juice
1 teaspoon grated orange rind
tarragon or parsley sprigs, to garnish
salt and pepper

1 Heat the oil in a heavy saucepan over a moderately high heat. Sauté the onion and potatoes for 2–3 minutes, or until the onions are translucent.

2 Add the tomatoes, tarragon, garlic, stock and salt and pepper to taste. Bring to the boil then reduce the heat and simmer, covered, for 20–25 minutes, or until the vegetables are tender.

3 Allow to cool slightly, then purée in a food processor or blender, then pass through a sieve and discard the pulp.

4 Stir the orange juice and rind into the soup. Reheat or serve chilled, garnished with tarragon or parsley sprigs.

# Chicken stock

alcohol free ✓  |  citrus free ✓  |  dairy free ✓  |  gluten free ✓  |  wheat free ✓

**Makes 1 litre (1¾ pints)**
**Preparation time: 5–10 minutes**
**Cooking time: 1¾ hours**

1.5 kg (3 lb) chicken
2.5 litres (4 pints) cold water
1 bouquet garni
small bunch of tarragon
1 small onion, stuck with 3 cloves
salt and pepper

**1** Put the chicken into a large saucepan with the water and bring
slowly to the boil. Remove any surface scum. Add the bouquet
garni, tarragon, the onion stuck with cloves and salt and pepper
to taste. Lower the heat and simmer gently for 1½ hours,
skimming regularly. Strain the stock through fine muslin or a very
fine strainer. Cool quickly and chill until required.

# Salads, vegetables and side dishes

## Wild rice, orange and walnut salad

alcohol free ✓  |  citrus free ✗  |  dairy free ✓  |  gluten free ✓  |  wheat free ✓

**Serves 4**
**Preparation time: 25 minutes**
**Cooking time: about 30 minutes**

**Per serving**
Energy 337 kcals/1407 kJ  |  Protein 8 g  |  Carbohydrate 56 g  |  Fat 9 g
Fibre 2 g

250 g (8 oz) wild rice
2 small oranges
1 small fennel bulb
3 spring onions, finely chopped
50 g (2 oz) walnut pieces
salt and pepper

**1** Bring a large saucepan of water to the boil. Add the wild rice, lower the heat and simmer for about 30 minutes or until tender. Drain the rice in a colander, refresh under cold running water, then drain thoroughly again. Transfer the cooked rice to a large salad bowl.

**2** Using a small sharp knife, peel away the skin and pith from the oranges. Slice them as thinly as possible and add to the rice. Trim the fennel bulb and reserve the fronds for garnish. Slice the fennel bulb and add to the salad bowl with the spring onions.

**3** Put the walnuts on a baking sheet and toast briefly under a preheated hot grill until they are lightly browned. Add to the salad, with salt and pepper to taste.

**4** To serve, sprinkle the salad with the reserved fennel fronds.

# Jersey royal and celery salad

alcohol free ✓ | citrus free ✕ | dairy free ✓ | gluten free ✓ | wheat free ✓

**Serves 4–6**
**Preparation time: 10 minutes, plus cooling**
**Cooking time: about 12 minutes**

**Per serving**
Energy 236 kcals/980 kJ | Protein 3 g | Carbohydrate 21 g | Fat 16 g
Fibre 3 g

500 g (1 lb) small Jersey Royal potatoes, scrubbed
6 celery sticks, with leaves if possible
75 g (3 oz) black olives
3 tablespoons capers, rinsed and drained
a few parsley sprigs, roughly chopped
1 quantity Tarragon and Lemon Dressing (see opposite)
salt and pepper

**1** Bring a saucepan of water to the boil. Add the potatoes and cook for about 12 minutes, until just tender. Drain in a colander and refresh under cold running water. Drain thoroughly once more and allow to cool.

**2** Slice the celery sticks diagonally and roughly chop any leaves. Place in a bowl with the olives, capers and parsley. Add the cooled potatoes and season with salt and pepper.

**3** Pour the dressing over the salad, toss well and serve.

# Tarragon and lemon dressing

alcohol free ✓ | citrus free ✕ | dairy free ✓ | gluten free ✓ | wheat free ✓

**Makes about 75 ml (3 fl oz)**
**Preparation time: 5 minutes**

**Per serving**
Energy 500 kcals/2065 kJ | Protein 1 g | Carbohydrate 1 g | Fat 55 g
Fibre 0 g

2 tablespoons tarragon vinegar
1 teaspoon finely grated lemon rind
¼ teaspoon Dijon mustard
1 tablespoon chopped tarragon
5 tablespoons olive oil or grapeseed oil
pinch of sugar
salt and pepper

**1** Combine the vinegar, lemon rind, mustard and tarragon in a
small bowl. Add the sugar and salt and pepper to taste. Stir to
mix, then gradually whisk in the oil, using a balloon whisk.
Alternatively, put all the ingredients in a screw-top jar, close
the lid tightly and shake well to combine.

# Grilled asparagus salad

alcohol free ✓ | citrus free ✗ | dairy free ✓ | gluten free ✓ | wheat free ✓

**Serves 4**
**Preparation time: 15 minutes**
**Cooking time: about 7 minutes**

**Per serving**
Energy 207 kcals/850 kJ | Protein 4 g | Carbohydrate 4 g | Fat 20 g
Fibre 2 g

500 g (1 lb) asparagus
3 tablespoons olive oil
about 50 g (2 oz) rocket
about 50 g (2 oz) lamb's lettuce
2 spring onions, finely chopped
3–4 radishes, thinly sliced
6 tablespoons Tarragon and Lemon Dressing (see page 179) or
   Classic French Dressing (see page 184)
salt and pepper

To Garnish:
roughly chopped herbs (such as tarragon, parsley, chervil and dill)
thin strips of lemon rind

**1** Trim the asparagus and use a potato peeler to peel about 5 cm
(2 inches) off the bottom of each stalk. Arrange in a single layer
on a baking sheet and brush with olive oil. Cook under a preheated hot grill for 7 minutes, turning until the asparagus spears
are just tender. Sprinkle with salt and pepper and leave to cool.

**2** Arrange the rocket and lamb's lettuce on a serving platter. Scatter
over the spring onions and radishes. Arrange the asparagus
beside the salad leaves and drizzle with the dressing. Garnish
with herbs and thin strips of lemon rind.

# Cucumber and dill salad

alcohol free ✓  |  citrus free ✓  |  dairy free ✗  |  gluten free ✓  |  wheat free ✓

**Serves 4–6**
**Preparation time: 15 minutes, plus standing**

**Per serving**
Energy 47 kcals/237 kJ  |  Protein 3 g  |  Carbohydrate 2 g  |  Fat 4 g
Fibre 0 g

1 cucumber, peeled and very thinly sliced
2 teaspoons salt
dill sprigs, to garnish

Dressing:
4 tablespoons thick natural yogurt or Greek yogurt
1 teaspoon white wine vinegar
2 tablespoons chopped dill
pepper

1 Put the cucumber slices in a colander, sprinkle with the salt and leave to stand for 20–30 minutes, to allow the excess moisture to drain away. Rinse the cucumber under cold running water, then drain thoroughly and place in a shallow serving dish.

2 To make the dressing, stir all the ingredients together in a small bowl.

3 Spoon the dressing over the cucumber and toss lightly to mix. Garnish with dill sprigs and serve.

# Butternut squash and wilted spinach salad

alcohol free ✓  |  citrus free ✗  |  dairy free ✓  |  gluten free ✓  |  wheat free ✓

**Serves 4–6**
**Preparation time: 15 minutes**
**Cooking time: 10 minutes**

**Per serving**

Energy 250 kcals/1040 kJ  |  Protein 4 g  |  Carbohydrate 17 g  |  Fat 19 g
Fibre 2 g

1 medium butternut squash, weighing about 750 g (1½ lb)
2 tablespoons extra-virgin olive oil
25 g (1 oz) pine nuts
175 g (6 oz) young spinach leaves
6 tablespoons of Classic French Dressing (see page 184) or Tarragon
  and Lemon Dressing (see page 179)
1 tablespoon chopped parsley
salt and pepper

1 Peel and slice the squash. Discard the seeds and cut the flesh into 1.5 cm (¾ inch) dice.

2 Add the squash to a pan of boiling water and cook for 4–5 minutes, until just tender. Drain thoroughly and refresh under cold running water, then drain again. Allow to cool.

3 Meanwhile, heat 1 tablespoon of the olive oil in a frying pan. Add the pine nuts and stir over a moderate heat for a minute or so, until they are golden brown. Transfer to a plate and set aside.

4 Add the remaining oil to the frying pan and return to the heat. Put in the spinach and stir for a few seconds until the leaves are just wilted. Remove from the heat.

5 Transfer the squash, pine nuts and spinach to a large shallow serving bowl. Toss all the ingredients lightly to mix well, and season with salt and pepper.

6 Mix together the dressing and parsley and spoon over the salad.

# Classic french dressing

alcohol free ✓ I citrus free ✓ I dairy free ✓ I gluten free ✓ I wheat free ✓

**Makes about 150 ml (¼ pint)**
**Preparation time: 5 minutes**

**Per serving**
Energy 627 kcals/2580 kJ I Protein 2 g I Carbohydrate 4 g I Fat 67 g
Fibre 0 g

2 tablespoons red or white vinegar
1–2 garlic cloves, crushed
2 teaspoons Dijon mustard
¼ teaspoon caster sugar
6 tablespoons olive oil
salt and pepper

**1** Combine the vinegar, garlic, mustard and sugar in a small bowl.
Add salt and pepper and stir well.

**2** Gradually whisk in the olive oil. Taste and add more salt and
pepper, if necessary. Alternatively, put all the ingredients in a
screw-top jar, close the lid tightly and shake well until combined.
Use as required.

# Mushroom, courgette and tomato salad

alcohol free ✓ | citrus free ✗ | dairy free ✓ | gluten free ✓ | wheat free ✓

**Serves 4**
**Preparation time: 10 minutes**

**Per serving**
Energy 47 kcals/200 kJ | Protein 3 g | Carbohydrate 8 g | Fat 1 g
Fibre 2 g

6 large mushrooms, sliced
4 courgettes, thinly sliced
4 tomatoes, skinned and quartered
1 tablespoon chopped basil
1 bunch of cress, trimmed and divided into sprigs
Citrus Dressing (see page 188), to serve

**1** Combine the mushrooms, courgettes and tomatoes in a salad
bowl and sprinkle with the basil.

**2** Arrange the sprigs of cress round the edge of the salad. Serve
with citrus dressing.

# Caponata

alcohol free ✓ I citrus free ✓ I dairy free ✓ I gluten free ✓ I wheat free ✓

**Serves 6**
**Preparation time: 20–30 minutes, plus draining**
**Cooking time: 1¼ hours**

**Per serving**
Energy 95 kcals/398 kJ I Protein 3 g I Carbohydrate 7 g I Fat 6 g
Fibre 5 g

3 aubergines cut into 1 cm (½ inch) dice
2 tablespoons olive oil
1 onion, thickly sliced
2 celery sticks, diced
150 ml (¼ pint) passata
3 tablespoons wine vinegar
1 yellow pepper, cored, deseeded and thinly sliced
1 red pepper, cored, deseeded and thinly sliced
25 g (1 oz) anchovy fillets, soaked in warm water, drained and dried
50 g (2 oz) capers, roughly chopped
25 g (1 oz) black olives, pitted and sliced
25 g (1 oz) green olives, pitted and sliced
salt
2 tablespoons chopped parsley, to serve

**1** Put the diced aubergines into a colander, sprinkle with salt and leave to drain for 15–20 minutes to exude their bitter juices. Rinse under cold running water to remove any salt and pat dry with kitchen paper.

**2** Heat the oil in a saucepan, add the onion and sauté until soft and golden. Add the celery and cook for 2–3 minutes. Add the aubergine and cook gently for 3 minutes, stirring occasionally. Add the passata and cook gently until it has been absorbed. Add the wine vinegar and cook for 1 minute. Add the peppers, anchovies, capers and olives and cook for 3 minutes.

**3** Transfer the mixture to an ovenproof dish and bake, covered, in a preheated oven, 180°C (350°F), Gas Mark 4, for about 1 hour. Serve lukewarm or cold sprinkled with chopped parsley.

# Citrus dressing

alcohol free ✓ I citrus free ✗ I dairy free ✓ I gluten free ✓ I wheat free ✓

**Makes about 125 ml (4 fl oz)**
**Preparation time: 5 minutes**

**Per serving**
Energy 40 kcals/170 kJ I Protein 1 g I Carbohydrate 10 g I Fat 0 g
Fibre 0 g

100 ml (3½ fl oz) orange juice
2 tablespoons lime juice
1 tablespoon lemon juice
1 teaspoon cider vinegar
½ teaspoon granular low-calorie sweetener
pepper

**1** Put all the ingredients into a screw-top jar and shake well.

# Stir-fried vegetables

alcohol free ✓ | citrus free ✓ | dairy free ✓ | gluten free ✓ | wheat free ✓

**Serves 4**
**Preparation time: 15–20 minutes**
**Cooking time: 3–5 minutes**

**Per serving**
Energy 66 kcals/275 kJ | Protein 3 g | Carbohydrate 7 g | Fat 3 g
Fibre 3 g

1 tablespoon vegetable oil
125 g (4 oz) bamboo shoots, thinly sliced
50 g (2 oz) mangetout
125 g (4 oz) carrots, thinly sliced
50 g (2 oz) broccoli florets
125 g (4 oz) fresh bean sprouts, rinsed
1 teaspoon each salt and sugar
1 tablespoon stock or water (optional)

**1** Heat the oil in a preheated wok or frying pan. Add the bamboo
shoots, mangetout, carrots and broccoli florets and stir-fry for
about 1 minute.

**2** Add the bean sprouts with the salt and sugar. Stir-fry for another
minute or so, then add some stock or water if necessary. Do not
overcook or the vegetables will lose their crunchiness. Serve hot.

# Main meals

## Peperonata with wholemeal noodles

alcohol free ✓ I citrus free ✓ I dairy free ✓ I gluten free ✕ I wheat free ✕

**Serves 6**
**Preparation time: 20–25 minutes**
**Cooking time: 20 minutes**

**Per serving**
Energy 170 kcals/720 kJ I Protein 6 g I Carbohydrate 28 g I Fat 5 g
Fibre ??g

2 tablespoons olive oil
1 large onion, thinly sliced
1 large garlic clove, crushed
2 red peppers, cored, deseeded and cut into strips
2 green peppers, cored, deseeded and cut into strips
375 g (12 oz) tomatoes, skinned, deseeded and chopped
1 tablespoon chopped basil
175 g (6 oz) wholemeal noodles
salt and pepper
basil sprigs, to garnish (optional)

**1** Heat 1 tablespoon of the olive oil in a deep frying pan. Add the onion and garlic and cook very gently until the onion is soft but not coloured. Add the peppers, tomatoes, basil and salt and pepper to taste. Cover and cook gently for 10 minutes.

**2** Remove the lid from the pan and cook over a fairly high heat until most of the liquid has evaporated. Keep the vegetable mixture warm.

**3** Meanwhile, cook the noodles in plenty of boiling salted water until just tender. Drain the noodles thoroughly and toss in the remaining olive oil. Add salt and pepper to taste.

**4** Divide the noodles among 4 serving plates and spoon the hot peperonata over the top. Garnish with basil sprigs and serve immediately.

# Seafood risotto

alcohol free ✓  |  citrus free ✓  |  dairy free ✕  |  gluten free ✓  |  wheat free ✓

**Serves 4**
**Preparation time: 15 minutes**
**Cooking time: about 35 minutes**

**Per serving**
Energy 490 kcals/2065 kJ  |  Protein 34 g  |  Carbohydrate 64 g  |  Fat 13 g
Fibre 4 g

50 g (2 oz) butter
1 onion, chopped
1 yellow pepper, cored, deseeded and chopped
1 red pepper, cored, deseeded and chopped
4 tomatoes, skinned, deseeded and chopped
375 g (12 oz) cod, skinned and cut into bite-sized pieces
8 scallops, cleaned
250 g (8 oz) medium-grain rice
475 ml (16 fl oz) hot stock
salt and pepper

To Garnish:
1 tablespoon finely chopped parsley
2 tablespoons freshly grated Parmesan cheese

1 Melt half the butter in a large heavy-based saucepan, add the onion, peppers and tomatoes, and fry gently for 1 minute, stirring occasionally.

2 Add the cod and scallops to the saucepan and fry for a further 3 minutes. Transfer to a bowl with a slotted spoon and season to taste with salt and pepper.

3 Melt the remaining butter in the pan, add the rice and fry for 3 minutes, stirring. Stir in the stock and 1 teaspoon salt. Bring to the boil, lower the heat and cover. Simmer for 15 minutes until the rice is almost tender and the liquid has been absorbed.

4 Gently stir the cod and scallop mixture into the rice and cook for 2 minutes to heat through.

5 Transfer to a warmed serving dish. Garnish with the parsley and sprinkle with the Parmesan.

# Spaghetti with three herb sauce

alcohol free ✕ | citrus free ✓ | dairy free ✓ | gluten free ✕ | wheat free ✕

**Serves 4**
**Preparation time: 15 minutes**
**Cooking time: 10–12 minutes**

**Per serving**
Energy 354 kcals/1500 kJ | Protein 12 g | Carbohydrate 70 g | Fat 5 g
Fibre 5 g

3 tablespoons chopped parsley
1 tablespoon chopped tarragon
2 tablespoons chopped basil
1 tablespoon olive oil
1 large garlic clove, crushed
4 tablespoons Chicken Stock (see page 175)
2 tablespoons dry white wine
375 g (12 oz) tricoloured spaghetti
salt and pepper

1 Put the parsley, tarragon, basil, olive oil, garlic, chicken stock and white wine into a food processor or blender with salt and pepper to taste and work until smooth.

2 Cook the spaghetti in a large pan of boiling salted water for 10–12 minutes until just tender.

3 Drain the spaghetti and heap in a warmed bowl. Pour over the herb sauce and toss well. Serve immediately.

# Pork casserole

alcohol free ✓ | citrus free ✓ | dairy free ✓ | gluten free ✓ | wheat free ✓

**Serves 4**
**Preparation time: 10 minutes**
**Cooking time: 35–40 minutes**

**Per serving**
Energy 300 kcals/1260 kJ | Protein 24 g | Carbohydrate 35 g | Fat 8 g
Fibre 6 g

375 g (12 oz) lean pork, diced
1 onion, sliced
150 g (5 oz) carrots, sliced
500 g (1 lb) baby new potatoes
400 ml (14 fl oz) pork stock
2 bay leaves
125 g (4 oz) frozen peas
75 g (3 oz) green beans, trimmed
25 g (1 oz) cornflour
50 ml (2 fl oz) cold water
pepper

**1** Trim any visible fat from the pork. Place the meat in a saucepan with the onion, carrots, potatoes, stock and bay leaves. Bring to the boil, cover and simmer for about 30 minutes, or until the meat is tender.

**2** Add the peas and beans. Blend the cornflour with the water and stir into the casserole. Bring back to the boil, then cover and simmer for a further 5 minutes, stirring occasionally.

**3** To serve, remove the bay leaves and season with a grinding of pepper.

# Lemon chicken

alcohol free ✓ I citrus free ✕ I dairy free ✓ I gluten free ✓ I wheat free ✓

**Serves 4**
**Preparation time: 15 minutes**
**Cooking time: 30–35 minutes**

**Per serving**
Energy 155 kcals/650 kJ I Protein 17 g I Carbohydrate 11 g I Fat 5 g
Fibre 0 g

1 tablespoon olive oil
1 small onion, thinly sliced
4 boneless, skinless chicken breasts, about 75 g (3 oz) each
2 tablespoons chopped parsley
300 ml (½ pint) Chicken Stock (see page 179)
1 tablespoon clear honey
juice of 1 lemon
2 teaspoons cornflour
1 tablespoon water
rind of 1 lemon, cut into strips
salt and pepper

**1** Heat the oil in a large frying pan. Add the onion and fry for 3–4
minutes. Add the chicken breasts and fry until lightly browned
all over. Add the parsley, stock, honey, lemon juice and salt and
pepper to taste. Cover the pan and simmer for 20 minutes.

**2** Using a slotted spoon, remove the chicken breasts to a warmed
serving dish, and keep warm.

**3** Blend the cornflour and water to a smooth paste, stir in the hot
cooking liquid, then return to the pan. Stir over a gentle heat
until thickened. Add the lemon rind to the sauce and spoon
evenly over the chicken.

# Chicken and sweet pepper kebabs

alcohol free ✓ | citrus free ✓ | dairy free ✗ | gluten free ✓ | wheat free ✓

**Serves 4**
**Preparation time: 15 minutes, plus marinating**
**Cooking time: 20 minutes**

**Per serving**
Energy 220 kcals/924 kJ | Protein 21 g | Carbohydrate 10 g | Fat 11 g
Fibre 2 g

150 ml (¼ pint) natural yogurt
2 tablespoons virgin olive oil
2 garlic cloves, crushed
2 tablespoons chopped coriander
2 teaspoons ground cumin
8 skinned and boned chicken thighs, cut into large chunks
1 onion, cut into chunks
1 red pepper, cored, deseeded and cut into chunks
1 green pepper, cored, deseeded and cut into chunks
salt and pepper

1 Mix together the yogurt, oil, garlic, coriander and cumin in a
shallow dish with salt and pepper to taste. Add the chicken cubes
and stir well to mix. Cover and marinate at room temperature for
30–60 minutes.

2 Thread the chicken cubes on to kebab skewers, alternating them
with pieces of onion and red and green pepper.

3 Put the kebabs on the rack of a grill pan. Place under a preheated hot grill and cook, turning frequently, for 20 minutes or
until the chicken is tender when pierced with a skewer or fork.
Serve hot on a bed of saffron rice with a cucumber and coriander
raita, if you like.

# Coq au vin

alcohol free ✗ | citrus free ✓ | dairy free ✓ | gluten free ✓ | wheat free ✓

**Serves 4**
**Preparation time: 10 minutes, plus marinating**
**Cooking time: about 1 hour**

**Per serving**
Energy 290 kcals/1225 kJ | Protein 24 g | Carbohydrate 6 g | Fat 17 g
Fibre 2 g

4 boneless, skinless chicken pieces, about 175 g (6 oz) each
4 tablespoons brandy
250 g (8 oz) button onions
900 ml (1½ pints) Chicken Stock (see page 175)
250 g (8 oz) button mushrooms
chopped parsley, to garnish

Marinade:
1 garlic clove, crushed
150 ml (¼ pint) red wine vinegar
150 ml (¼ pint) red wine
1 tablespoon Worcestershire sauce
salt and pepper

**1** Combine all the marinade ingredients. Place the chicken pieces in a large shallow bowl and pour the marinade over them. Cover and set aside in a cool place for at least 3 hours, turning occasionally.

**2** Drain the chicken pieces, reserving the marinade, and brown briefly under a preheated grill. Transfer the chicken pieces to a casserole.

**3** Pour the brandy over the chicken and ignite. When the flames die down, add the onions and stock. Cover and cook in a preheated oven, 220°C (425°F), Gas Mark 7, for 50 minutes.

**4** Add the mushrooms and cook for 10 minutes, or until the chicken pieces are tender and the juices run clear when the thickest parts are pierced with a skewer.

**5** Meanwhile, pour the reserved marinade into a saucepan and boil rapidly, uncovered, until reduced by half. Stir into the casserole. Garnish with the chopped parsley and serve at once.

# Vegetable chow mein

alcohol free ✕ I citrus free ✓ I dairy free ✓ I gluten free ✕ I wheat free ✕

**Serves 4**
**Preparation time: 10–15 minutes**
**Cooking time: about 8 minutes**

**Per serving**
Energy 380 kcals/1606 kJ I Protein 12 g I Carbohydrate 62 g I Fat 11 g
Fibre 7 g

250 g (8 oz) dried thread or fine egg noodles
2 tablespoons groundnut oil
2 carrots, cut into matchsticks
1 green pepper, cored, deseeded and cut lengthways into thin strips
3 celery sticks, cut into matchsticks
200 g (7 oz) canned water chestnuts, drained and cut into
   matchsticks
175 g (6 oz) Chinese leaves, trimmed and shredded
175 g (6 oz) spinach, trimmed and shredded
salt and pepper

Sauce:
2 teaspoons cornflour
4 tablespoons cold water
2 tablespoons soy sauce
1 tablespoon rice wine or dry sherry

**1** For the sauce, blend the cornflour to a thin paste with the cold water, soy sauce and rice wine or sherry.

**2** Break the noodles into pieces with your hands, then cook them according to the packet instructions.

**3** Meanwhile, heat a wok. Add the oil and when hot add the carrots, pepper and celery and stir-fry for 2–3 minutes.

**4** Stir the sauce then pour it into the wok and bring to the boil, stirring constantly. Remove the wok from the heat.

**5** Drain the noodles and add them to the wok. Return the wok to a high heat, add the water chestnuts, Chinese leaves and spinach and toss for 1–2 minutes or until all the ingredients are combined and the spinach is just wilted. Add salt and pepper to taste and serve hot.

# Sole and smoked salmon paupiettes

alcohol free ✓ | citrus free ✗ | dairy free ✗ | gluten free ✓ | wheat free ✓

**Serves 6**
**Preparation time: 15 minutes**
**Cooking time: about 15 minutes**

**Per serving**
Energy 67 kcals/285 kJ | Protein 14 g | Carbohydrate 0 g | Fat 1 g
Fibre 0 g

6 small sole fillets, about 50 g (2 oz) each, skinned
3 slices smoked salmon, about 25 g (1 oz)
1 tablespoon chopped dill
300 ml (½ pint) fish stock
300 ml (½ pint) Herb and Lemon Sauce (see page 205), optional
50 g (2 oz) cooked peeled prawns
salt and pepper

To Garnish:
dill sprigs
lemon twists

1 Lay the sole fillets flat and season with salt and pepper. Cut the slices of smoked salmon in half lengthways and lay a strip down the length of each sole fillet. Sprinkle with chopped dill and roll up loosely. Secure with wooden cocktail sticks.

2 Place the fish rolls in a shallow pan and add the fish stock – it should cover the fish. Cover and simmer for about 8 minutes until just tender. Drain the fish and keep warm in a serving dish.

3 Spoon 4 tablespoons of the fish cooking liquid into a small pan and boil quickly over a high heat until reduced to about 1 tablespoon.

4 Stir the herb and lemon sauce, if using, and the prawns into the reduced cooking liquid and heat through gently. Spoon the sauce evenly over the fish paupiettes and garnish with dill sprigs and lemon twists.

# Stir-fried beef with peppers

alcohol free ✕ | citrus free ✓ | dairy free ✓ | gluten free ✕ | wheat free ✕

**Serves 6**
**Preparation time: 10 minutes**
**Cooking time: 10–12 minutes**

**Per serving**
Energy 159 kcals/663 kJ | Protein 18 g | Carbohydrate 4 g | Fat 7 g
Fibre 1 g

1 tablespoon olive oil
1 onion, thinly sliced
1 large garlic clove, cut into thin strips
500 g (1 lb) fillet steak, cut into thin strips
1 red pepper, cored, deseeded and cut into matchsticks
1 green pepper, cored, deseeded and cut into matchsticks
1 tablespoon soy sauce
2 tablespoons dry sherry
1 tablespoon chopped rosemary
salt and pepper
brown rice, to serve

**1** Heat the olive oil in a wok or deep frying pan and stir-fry the onion and garlic for 2 minutes.

**2** Add the strips of beef and stir-fry briskly until evenly browned on all sides and almost tender.

**3** Add the strips of pepper and stir-fry for 2 minutes.

**4** Add the soy sauce, sherry, rosemary and salt and pepper to taste and stir-fry for a further 1–2 minutes. Serve piping hot with brown rice.

# Herb and lemon sauce

alcohol free ✓ | citrus free ✕ | dairy free ✕ | gluten free ✓ | wheat free ✓

**Makes about 300 ml (½ pint)**
**Preparation time: 10 minutes**

**Per serving**
Energy 449 kcals/1863 kJ | Protein 15 g | Carbohydrate 19 g | Fat 35 g
Fibre 0 g

2 hard-boiled egg yolks
grated rind and juice of 1 lemon
1 teaspoon French mustard
1 teaspoon soft dark brown sugar
4 tablespoons vegetable stock
2 tablespoons olive oil
4 tablespoons natural yogurt
1 tablespoon each finely chopped tarragon, basil and parsley
salt and pepper

**1** Mix the egg yolks to a paste with the lemon rind and juice, mustard and sugar. Gradually beat in the stock, olive oil and yogurt then add the herbs and salt and pepper to taste.

# Vegetable hot pot

alcohol free ✓ | citrus free ✓ | dairy free ✓ | gluten free ✓ | wheat free ✓

**Serves 4**
**Preparation time: 10 minutes**
**Cooking time: about 25 minutes**

**Per serving**
Energy 155 kcals/655 kJ | Protein 5 g | Carbohydrate 31 g | Fat 2 g
Fibre 10 g

4 carrots, sliced
4 parsnips, sliced
2 large courgettes, sliced
2 turnips, sliced
2 red or green peppers, cored, deseeded and roughly chopped
2 onions, sliced
2 large tomatoes, skinned, deseeded and chopped
600 ml (1 pint) Chicken Stock (see page 175)
1 bay leaf
1 tablespoon chopped parsley
1 tablespoon chopped thyme
1 teaspoon chopped marjoram
dash of Worcestershire sauce
salt and pepper

**1** Place all the ingredients in a flameproof casserole. Bring to the
boil, skim off the scum, then cover and cook gently for about 25
minutes, until all the vegetables are tender. Serve the hotpot
immediately.

# Desserts

## Yogurt fruit cup

alcohol free ✓ | citrus free ✓ | dairy free ✗ | gluten free ✓ | wheat free ✓

**Serves 6**
**Preparation time: 10 minutes**

**Per serving**
Energy 114 kcals/483 kJ | Protein 4 g | Carbohydrate 21 g | Fat 2 g
Fibre 1 g

500 g (1 lb) can sliced peaches or pears in fruit juice, drained
475 ml (16 fl oz) low-fat vanilla yogurt
2 tablespoons finely chopped toasted almonds
½ teaspoon ground cardamom

**1** Divide the fruit among 6 small dessert bowls. Top with yogurt
and sprinkle lightly with almonds and cardamom. Serve
immediately.

# Melon ice cream

alcohol free ✓ | citrus free ✓ | dairy free ✗ | gluten free ✓ | wheat free ✓

**Serves 4**
**Preparation time: 20–25 minutes, plus freezing**

**Per serving**
Energy 94 kcals/397 kJ | Protein 5 g | Carbohydrate 17 g | Fat 1 g
Fibre 2 g

1 large melon (Ogen or Charentais)
300 ml (½ pint) natural yogurt

1 Halve the melon and scoop out all the seeds. Scoop the melon flesh into a food processor or blender and work until smooth.

2 Mix the melon purée with the yogurt. Transfer the melon and yogurt mixture to a shallow freezer container and freeze until firm.

3 Serve the melon ice cream in scoops.

# Coconut cookies

alcohol free ✓ | citrus free ✓ | dairy free ✓ | gluten free ✓ | wheat free ✓

**Makes 24 cookies**
**Preparation time: 10 minutes**
**Cooking time: 15–20 minutes**

**Per serving**
Energy 94 kcals/392 kJ | Protein 1 g | Carbohydrate 10 g | Fat 6 g
Fibre 1 g

125 g (4 oz) margarine or goat's butter
50 g (2 oz) golden syrup
50 g (2 oz) unrefined demerara sugar
1 level teaspoon bicarbonate of soda
50 g (2 oz) freshly grated or desiccated coconut
75 g (3 oz) millet flakes
125 g (4 oz) brown rice flour

**1** Put the margarine or butter, syrup and sugar into a large saucepan and stir over a low heat until the fat and sugar have melted. Remove from the heat, add the bicarbonate of soda and stir well to dissolve. (The mixture rises up the pan during this stage.) Add the rest of the ingredients and blend thoroughly.

**2** Cool slightly, then gather the mixture together and roll into about 24 balls.

**3** Put the balls on 2 greased baking sheets, allowing plenty of space for the mixture to spread out during cooking.

**4** Bake in a preheated oven, 160°C (325°F), Gas Mark 3, for 15–20 minutes or until golden brown. Leave the cookies on the baking sheets until almost cold, then transfer to a wire rack to cool completely.

# Peach crisp

alcohol free ✓  |  citrus free ✗  |  dairy free ✗  |  gluten free ✗  |  wheat free ✓

**Serves 6–8**
**Preparation time: 15 minutes**
**Cooking time: 25–30 minutes**

**Per serving**
Energy 337 kcals/ 1407kJ  |  Protein 4 g  |  Carbohydrate 50 g  |  Fat 15 g
Fibre 6 g

1.5 kg (3 lb) peaches, skinned, stoned and thickly sliced
2 teaspoons lemon juice
25 g (1 oz) flour
3 tablespoons dry breadcrumbs
40 g (1½ oz) quick-cook oatmeal
125 g (4 oz) light brown sugar
½ teaspoon ground cinnamon
¼ teaspoon each grated nutmeg and ground ginger
100 g (3½ oz) butter

**1** Mix the peaches with the lemon juice and place in a well-greased 2 litre (1¾ pint) shallow ovenproof dish.

**2** In a mixing bowl, combine the flour, breadcrumbs, oatmeal, sugar and spices with the butter and crumble together. Sprinkle the mixture evenly over the peaches and pat down lightly.

**3** Bake in a preheated oven, 190°C (375°F), Gas Mark 5, for 25–30 minutes until browned and crusty on top. Serve with vanilla ice cream or whipped cream, if liked.

# Glossary

**COLITIS** Inflammation of the colon, or large intestine. The term may be used to refer to any of a number of disorders involving the colon. Symptoms include diarrhoea (often with blood and mucus), abdominal pain, and fever.

**ENZYMES** A group of proteins that speed up certain biochemical reactions.

**FIBROMYALGIA** A condition characterized by muscular aches, pains and stiffness. Fibromyalgia is often accompanied by fatigue.

**FUNCTIONAL BOWEL DISORDERS** A description which encompasses IBS and other conditions when the way in which the bowel works has altered.

**GASTROINTESTINAL**  Relating to the intestines and stomach.

**HOLISTIC**  Treatment of the whole body rather than specific parts.

**MALABSORPTION**  Difficulty in the digestion or absorption of nutrients from food substances.

**METABOLISM**  The sum of all biochemical processes involved in life. Exercise, food and environmental temperature all influence metabolism.

**MOTILITY**  The muscular activity of the gut.

**NON-STEROIDAL ANTI- INFLAMMATORIES**  These suppress inflammation in a manner similar to steroids, but without the side effects. They are also used for alleviating pain and fever.

**PERISTALSIS**  Involuntary muscle contractions that move waste matter through the alimentary tract.

**PORPHYRIA**  A disorder in which the body produces too much of the chemical porphyrin. It is an inherited condition.

**PROSTAGLANDIN**  These substances are not stored but are produced as needed in nearly every body tissue. They have been found to regulate smooth muscle activity.

**SEROTONIN**  An adult human contains about 5 to 10 mg of serotonin, most of which is in the intestine and the rest in blood platelets and the brain. One of its functions is as a neurotransmitter which affects learning, sleep and mood.

**SOMATIZATION** A physical manifestation of emotional disorders.

# General index

# Recipe index